T0249427

Radiculopathy

Guest Editor

DAVID J. KENNEDY, MD

PHYSICAL MEDICINE AND REHABILITATION CLINICS OF NORTH AMERICA

www.pmr.theclinics.com

Consulting Editor
GEORGE H. KRAFT, MD, MS

February 2011 • Volume 22 • Number 1

SAUNDERS an imprint of ELSEVIER, Inc.

W.B. SAUNDERS COMPANY
A Division of Elsevier Inc.

1600 John F. Kennedy Boulevard • Suite 1800 • Philadelphia, Pennsylvania 19103

http://www.theclinics.com

PHYSICAL MEDICINE AND REHABILITATION CLINICS OF NORTH AMERICA Volume 22, Number 1
February 2011 ISSN 1047-9651, ISBN-13: 978-1-4557-0490-3

Editor: Debora Dellapena

Reprints. For copies of 100 or more of articles in this publication, please contact the Commercial Reprints Department, Elsevier Inc., 360 Park Avenue South, New York, NY 10010-1710. Tel.: 212-633-3812; Fax: 212-462-1935; E-mail: reprints@elsevier.com.

Physical Medicine and Rehabilitation Clinics of North America (ISSN 1047-9651) is published quarterly by Elsevier Inc., 360 Park Avenue South, New York, NY 10010-1710. Months of issue are February, May, August, and November. Business and Editorial Offices: 1600 John F. Kennedy Blvd., Suite 1800, Philadelphia, PA 19103-2899. Customer Service Office: 3251 Riverport Lane, Maryland Heights, MO 63043. Periodicals postage paid at New York, NY and additional mailing offices. Subscription price per year is $230.00 (US individuals), $414.00 (US institutions), $122.00 (US students), $280.00 (Canadian individuals), $540.00 (Canadian institutions), $175.00 (Canadian students), $345.00 (foreign individuals), $540.00 (foreign institutions), and $175.00 (foreign students). Foreign air speed delivery is included in all *Clinics* subscription prices. All prices are subject to change without notice. **POSTMASTER:** Send address changes to *Physical Medicine and Rehabilitation Clinics of North America*, Customer Service Office: Elsevier Health Sciences Division, Subscription Customer Service, 3251 Riverport Lane, Maryland Heights, MO 63043. **Customer Service: 1-800-654-2452 (US). From outside of the United States, call 314-447-8871. Fax: 314-447-8029. E-mail: JournalsCustomer Service-usa@elsevier.com (for print support); JournalsOnlineSupport-usa@elsevier.com (for online support).**

Physical Medicine and Rehabilitation Clinics of North America is indexed in *Excerpta Medica, MEDLINE/ PubMed (Index Medicus), Cinahl,* and *Cumulative Index to Nursing and Allied Health Literature.*

Printed and bound by CPI Group (UK) Ltd, Croydon, CR0 4YY

Transferred to Digital Print 2011

Contributors

CONSULTING EDITOR

GEORGE H. KRAFT, MD, MS
Alvord Professor of Multiple Sclerosis Research; Professor, Department of Rehabilitation Medicine and Adjunct Professor, Department of Neurology, University of Washington School of Medicine, Seattle, Washington

GUEST EDITOR

DAVID J. KENNEDY, MD
Assistant Professor, Associate Fellowship Director Physical Medicine and Rehabilitation Spine and Musculoskeletal Fellowship, Department of Orthopaedics and Rehabilitation, University of Florida College of Medicine, Gainesville, Florida

AUTHORS

GERT BRONFORT, PhD, DC
Vice President of Research, Wolfe-Harris Center for Clinical Studies, Northwestern Health Sciences University, Bloomington, Minnesota

ADAM J. BRUGGEMAN, MD
Resident, Department of Orthopaedics and Rehabilitation, University of Florida, Gainesville, Florida

ELLEN CASEY, MD
Attending Physician, Clinical Instructor, Sports and Spine Rehabilitation, Rehabilitation Institute of Chicago, Northwestern University Feinberg School of Medicine, Chicago, Illinois

DAVID S. CHENG, MD
Department of Rehabilitation and Regenerative Medicine, Columbia University College of Physicians and Surgeons, New York, New York

ROBERT C. DECKER, MD
Assistant Professor, Department of Orthopaedics and Rehabilitation, Orthopaedics and Sports Medicine Institute, University of Florida, Gainesville, Florida

ARTHUR J. DE LUIGI, DO
Assistant Professor of Neurology, Uniformed Services University of Health Sciences, Bethesda, Maryland; Program Director, Physical Medicine and Rehabilitation Residency; Assistant Chief, Physical Medicine and Rehabilitation Service, Department of Orthopaedics and Rehabilitation, Walter Reed Army Medical Center, Washington, DC

RONALD DONELSON, MD, MS
President, SelfCare First, LLC, Hanover, New Hampshire

RONI EVANS, MS, DC
Dean of Research, Wolfe-Harris Center for Clinical Studies, Northwestern Health Sciences University, Bloomington, Minnesota

KEVIN F. FITZPATRICK, MD
Director, Physical Medicine and Rehabilitation Residency; Associate Program Director, Electrodiagnostic Medicine, Department of Orthopaedics and Rehabilitation, Walter Reed Army Medical Center, Washington, DC; Assistant Professor of Neurology, Uniformed Services University of Health Sciences, Bethesda, Maryland

ANAND B. JOSHI, MD, MHA
Clinical Instructor, Penn Spine Center, Department of Physical Medicine and Rehabilitation, University of Pennsylvania, Philadelphia, Pennsylvania

DAVID J. KENNEDY, MD
Assistant Professor, Department of Orthopaedics and Rehabilitation, University of Florida College of Medicine, Gainesville, Florida

BRENT LEININGER, DC
Research Fellow, Wolfe-Harris Center for Clinical Studies, Northwestern Health Sciences University, Bloomington, Minnesota

JOSE MENA, MD
Assistant Professor, Department of Rehabilitation Medicine, University of Miami Miller School of Medicine, Miami, Florida

MAUREEN Y. NOH, MD
Physical Medicine and Rehabilitation Spine and Musculoskeletal Fellow, Department of Orthopaedics and Rehabilitation, University of Florida, Gainesville, Florida

CHRISTOPHER T. PLASTARAS, MD
Director, Penn Spine Center, Department of Physical Medicine and Rehabilitation, University of Pennsylvania, Philadelphia, Pennsylvania

TODD REITER, MD, DC
Medical Director, Inpatient Rehabilitation Center, High Point Regional Health System, High Point, North Carolina

MONICA E. RHO, MD
Clinical Instructor, Department of Physical Medicine and Rehabilitation, Northwestern University Feinberg School of Medicine/Rehabilitation Institute of Chicago, Chicago, Illinois

ANDREW L. SHERMAN, MD
Associate Professor and Vice-Chair, Department of Rehabilitation Medicine, University of Miami Miller School of Medicine, Miami, Florida

ALISON STOUT, DO
Director, Spine and Musculoskeletal Medicine, Rehabilitation Care Services, Veterans Administration, Puget Sound; Acting Assistant Professor, Department of Rehabilitation, University of Washington, Seattle, Washington

CHI-TSAI TANG, MD
Clinical Instructor, Department of Orthopaedic Surgery, Division of Physical Medicine and Rehabilitation, Washington University School of Medicine, Washington University Orthopedics, St Louis, Missouri

CHRISTOPHER J. VISCO, MD
Assistant Professor of Clinical Rehabilitation, Department of Rehabilitation and Regenerative Medicine, Columbia University College of Physicians and Surgeons, New York, New York

Contents

> Radicular pain is a frequent complaint of patients presenting to outpatient primary care and musculoskeletal clinics. Most cases of radiculopathy are self-limiting, and symptoms resolve over the course of weeks to months. There is spontaneous resolution of disc herniations, and clinical improvement correlates with morphologic resolution. Knowledge of the natural history of radiculopathy is crucial for the health care provider to appropriately counsel and treat patients with this disorder. Although each patient should be managed individually, the favorable prognosis of radiculopathy based on the natural history supports a conservative approach for the initial weeks to months for most patients.

> History and physical examination is the cornerstone in the appropriate diagnosis and treatment of any patient. A comprehensive physical examination is necessary to aid in determining distributions of symptoms and to lead one to the site of pathology. The aim of this article is to aid the clinician in distinguishing radiculopathy from other causes of neck and low back pain. Physical examination of the patient with suspected radiculopathy needs to be thorough and complete to make the most accurate diagnosis. Thorough knowledge of the evidence-based literature is beneficial in maximizing patient care, particularly in the light of health care reform.

> All patients presenting with signs and symptoms of lumbar radiculopathy must undergo a thorough history taking and physical examination. Often, however, the diagnosis remains unclear; it is accurate anatomically, but the underlying cause of the lesion is not confirmed, or the symptoms are so severe that more information on the anatomy is required. Therefore, the next step in the diagnostic process is imaging studies. This article discusses imaging modalities, including plain radiographs, magnetic resonance imaging, computed tomography (CT), CT myelogram, selective nerve root block, and bone scan.

Pharmaceutical treatments for radiculopathy include opioid, antiinflammatory (steroidal and nonsteroidal), neuromodulating, topical, and adjuvant treatments. These medications act locally, peripherally, or centrally on the neural axis. This article reviews the history of medication use for radiculopathy and the available literature along with the breadth of current treatment and indications.

Conservative management of low back pain includes the use of lumbar epidural steroid injections, which have become increasingly more popular in the last 20 years. The body of literature regarding the efficacy of these injections is vast, conflicting, and difficult to summarize. This article reviews the updated evidence for efficacy and the indications for these injections.

Epidural steroid injection (ESI) has been used to treat cervical radiculopathy for several decades. Generally, available studies demonstrate favorable results, although definitive evidence of efficacy is lacking. ESIs are not considered a first line treatment and are undertaken after non-interventional treatments have been adequately provided. In the cervical spine, where evidence of potential benefit is moderate and there is risk of major complication, non-interventional care is even more germane. This article reviews the available literature regarding risks and efficacy of ESIs for cervical radiculopathy, and aims to guide practitioners in treatment decisions for individual patients.

Lumbar disk herniation is a significant cause of lumbar radiculopathy and results in billions of dollars in health care expenditure. Herniated lumbar disks cause mechanical and chemical irritation of the nerve roots leading to complaints of sciatica. Surgeons have several surgical options when approaching herniated disks, including various microsurgical procedures. The 3 most prominent studies to date on surgical and nonsurgical management of herniated disks agree on the efficacy of surgery over medical management in the short term but have some discrepancies when looking at long-term results. Cauda equina syndrome is a variation of lumbar disk herniation in which patients experience a combination of saddle anesthesia, abnormal lower extremity reflexes, and neurogenic bowel or bladder symptoms.

THE CLINICS ARE NOW AVAILABLE ONLINE!

Access your subscription at:
www.theclinics.com

Foreword

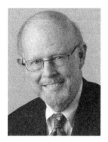

George H. Kraft, MD, MS
Consulting Editor

Over the years that *Physical Medicine and Rehabilitation Clinics of North America* has been published, there has been a change in interests of new practitioners in the field of PM&R. From my perspective, I see this as a phase of a longer series of cycles, encompassing much of the last 100 years.

These sinusoidal cycles consist of musculoskeletal medicine (MSK), "sports and spine," or some other version of anato-kinesiologically based medical care as one phase alternating with a more neurophysiologically based practice as the other. These phases are decades long. When I did my residency training in the late 1960s, the field was shifting from the MSK phase to the "neuro" phase. That shifted back and I feel that we have now been in the MSK phase for between 10 and 15 years. By any measure, we now appear to substantially well into the MSK phase, with between 50% and 70% of our residency graduates currently opting for this type of practice.

Let us take a moment and look back to the MSK phase before the phase shift to neuro in the late 1960s. This MSK phase began around 1930-1935 and was based on the putative healing powers of the various physical modalities that were developed around this time. Diathermy and massage were widely used and did indeed reduce the discomfort of MSK pain.

To summarize, in its infancy in the 1930s, the field of PM&R was MSK-based, relying largely on the modalities for treatments. In the 1960s there was a phase shift to neuro-based practice. Then from the 1990s on, a shift back to MSK practice occurred.

Of course it is not quite this simple. There is also the effect on the field of the tension between outpatient and inpatient practice; outpatient care favors MSK management, whereas inpatient care favors neuro-rehabilitation (eg, spinal cord injury). There is the tension between academia, favoring inpatient care, and private practice favoring outpatient care. Finally, there are the final echoes of the "big bang" between the Krusian concept (Frank Krusen, MD, founder of the Department of Physical Medicine at the Mayo Clinic, mostly outpatient-based) and Ruskian concept (Howard Rusk, MD, founder of the Department of Rehabilitation Medicine at New York University, mostly inpatient-based). Does this help explain why our field of practice still has two names: physical medicine and rehabilitation?

Phys Med Rehabil Clin N Am 22 (2011) xi–xii
doi:10.1016/j.pmr.2010.12.003
1047-9651/11/$ – see front matter © 2011 Elsevier Inc. All rights reserved.

pmr.theclinics.com

Although history is interesting in and of itself, there are also practical reasons we study it: we can learn from it. A very important lesson is to learn why modality outpatient practice was abandoned after its initial 30-year phase. Although modalities made patients feel better, their efficacy was not substantiated and other improved treatments were developed.

That is one of my concerns about the current MSK phase: many of the expensive MSK procedures done in practice have not been proven effective by random, controlled trials. Because they are very effective in bringing in revenue, there is pressure on practitioners to do them. But as the blanket of universal health care coverage settles over the nation, running headlong into the competing mandate to reduce the federal deficit, it is difficult for an observer to believe that serious scrutiny will not be given to expensive, but still unproven, health care.

It is really heartening to see the list of young MSK academicians who Dr Kennedy has assembled as contributors to this issue. I know many of them and think very highly of them as academic MSK physiatrists, who understand the importance of determining the scientific merit of their art. I have confidence in the Guest Editor's choices that those whom I don't personally know have the same dedication to academic medicine. In reviewing the 12 articles it is apparent that the assessment and nonsurgical management of radiculopathies have been comprehensively addressed. Knowing D. J. Kennedy as I do, the reader can be assured that this issue is packed with accurate and useful up-to-date information on caring for patients with cervical and lumbosacral radicular symptoms. I hope that the reader will concur with this assessment.

George H. Kraft, MD, MS
Department of Rehabilitation Medicine
University of Washington
1959 NE Pacific Street, RJ-30
Seattle, WA 98195, USA

E-mail address:
ghkraft@uw.edu

Preface

Radiculopathy

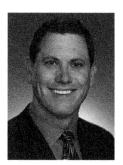

David J. Kennedy, MD
Guest Editor

It is with great honor that we present this edition of the *Physical Medicine and Rehabilitation Clinics of North America* on Radiculopathy. This is one of the few medical conditions that truly acts as a "cross cutting" topic and in doing so spans the field of Physical Medicine and Rehabilitation. While it is a mainstay of the musculoskeletal specialist, it is our background in neurologic training that truly makes the Physical Medicine and Rehabilitation physician so adept at both diagnosing and treating radiculopathy. A thorough understanding of the nervous system, including dermatomes, myotomes, and electordiagnosis, is essential to obtaining an accurate diagnosis. This, combined with our knowledge of manipulation, mechanical therapy, anatomy and muscle activation patterns, medications, and invasive treatments, allows the practitioner to implement the best possible treatment algorithm for our patients.

This edition is presented in a systematic manner, one which mimics the clinical encounter and treatment pathways. It starts with natural history and physical examination and is followed by diagnostic studies including imaging and electrodiagnostics. Noninvasive treatment may include some combination of mechanical therapy, manipulation, and/or core stability. For more severe or refractory cases, medications, injections, or even surgery may be required.

These articles serve as a comprehensive and up-to-date review of all of these topics. I want to once again thank the authors (Casey, De Luigi, Fitzpatrick, Mena, Sherman, Plastaras, Joshi, Donelson, Noh, Leininger, Bronfort, Evans, Reiter, Visco, Cheng, Rho, Tang, Stout, Bruggeman, and Decker) for their tireless work, expertise, and enthusiasm as they devoted their valuable time and thought in creating this edition.

Phys Med Rehabil Clin N Am 22 (2011) xiii–xiv
doi:10.1016/j.pmr.2010.12.004

I cannot overstate how honored I was to work with all of them and be the Guest Editor for this issue. I hope you find this resource both informative and practical.

David J. Kennedy, MD
Department of Orthopaedics and Rehabilitation
University of Florida College of Medicine
c/o Marlene Gardner
4101 NW 89th Boulevard
Gainesville, FL 32606, USA

E-mail address:
djkennedy@gmail.com

Natural History of Radiculopathy

Ellen Casey, MD

KEYWORDS

• Radiculopathy • Radicular pain • Natural history

Approximately two-thirds of adults suffer from neck and low back pain.[1] Axial spine pain is often accompanied by radicular pain or radiculopathy, which is defined as spinal nerve root dysfunction causing dermatomal pain and parasthesias, myotomal weakness, and/or impaired deep tendon reflexes. Mixer and Barr first introduced the concept of herniated disc material leading to radiculopathy in 1934.[2] Since that landmark study, extensive research has been conducted on the pathogenesis, clinical presentation, and treatment of radiculopathy. An understanding of the natural history of radiculopathy is crucial because it better enables health care providers to counsel patients, recommend treatments, and assess outcomes of specific interventions. Although it can be challenging to sort through the available information given the vast differences in diagnostic criteria, length of follow-up periods, and exposure of many patients to some type of conservative management, this article aims to combine the findings from several landmark papers to provide a concise summary of the natural evolution of radiculopathy.

EPIDEMIOLOGY

The estimated prevalence of radiculopathy is 9.8 per 1000 and 3.5 cases per 1000 in the lumbosacral and cervical spine, respectively.[3,4] Patients with lumbosacral radiculopathy tend to present in the late 1920s to 1940s, whereas the peak age of presentation for cervical radiculopathy is in the sixth decade.[5,6] Various risk factors have been investigated for a causative role in the development of radiculopathy, including gender, prior episodes of neck or back pain, and occupational or recreational factors. Although some studies suggest that radiculopathy occurs more frequently in men, others have shown equal rates between genders.[5–7] Previous history of axial low back pain is a well-established risk factor for lumbosacral radiculopathy, and a prior history of lumbosacral radiculopathy has been found in patients presenting with cervical radiculopathy. Additionally, prior history of trauma was found in approximately 15% of cases of cervical radiculopathy but this association has not been documented in the

The author has nothing to disclose.
Sports & Spine Rehabilitation, Rehabilitation Institute of Chicago/Northwestern University Feinberg School of Medicine, 1030 North Clark Street, Suite 500, Chicago, IL 60610, USA
E-mail address: ecasey@ric.org

doi:10.1016/j.pmr.2010.10.001
1047-9651/11/$ – see front matter © 2011 Elsevier Inc. All rights reserved.

lumbar spine. Although there is a correlation between a higher body mass and low back pain, the same relationship does not appear to exist in radiculopathy.[7] Multiple studies have shown a genetic linkage for spinal canal size as well as occurrence of disc herniation and subsequent radiculopathy.[8–10] In regards to occupational factors, lumbosacral radiculopathy occurs more frequently in patients who have performed jobs requiring manual labor, and who work in positions of sustained lumbar flexion or rotation and who engage in prolonged driving.[11–13]

NATURAL HISTORY
Lumbosacral Radiculopathy

The first study to follow the clinical course of patients with lumbosacral radiculopathy was written by Hakelius[14] in 1970. Of the 38 patients with a clinical presentation consistent with radiculopathy and a disc herniation demonstrated on myelography, 88% reported that they were *symptom-free* after 6 months. In 1983, Weber[7] published a paper documenting a prospective study of 126 patients with "sciatica". These patients were randomized to surgery or conservative management and followed for 10 years. The primary treatment given to the 66 patients in the conservative group was bed rest and paracetamol. Some patients also received physical therapy, but the type and frequency was not documented. Sixty-seven percent of patients in the conservative group reported good to fair outcomes at 1 year, 4 years and 10 years. Saal and Saal[15] conducted another prospective study that was published in 1989. They followed 58 patients with a diagnosis of radiculopathy based on physical exam-ination, imaging, and electrodiagnostic testing. The patients were exposed to minimal treatment, including back school and stabilization exercises. At the conclusion of the 31-week follow-up period, 92% reported a good to excellent outcome and 92% had returned to work. Another paper by Weber and colleagues [16] focused on the short-term evolution of lumbosacral radiculopathy in 208 patients. These patients were placed on bed rest for one week, and then allowed to gradually resume activity. None of the patients underwent physical therapy. After 4 weeks, 70% of patients had marked reduction in pain, which corresponded to functional improvement, and 60% had returned to work. Weber's studies have also investigated prognostic risk factors of recovery as well as recurrence. The factors that correlated with a poor outcome or prolonged recovery included female gender, psychosocial problems, greater than 3 months sick leave before presentation, and a prior history of radiculop-athy. A recurrence of symptoms occurs in approximately 20% of patients.[7,16]

Cervical Radiculopathy

The course of clinical improvement of cervical radiculopathy is even less well docu-mented than that of lumbosacral radiculopathy. Spurling and Segerberg[17] published one of the first papers that attempted to address this question in 1953. They followed 110 patients with cervical radiculopathy who were primarily treated with 7 to 10 days of bed rest and traction. The average follow-up period was 23 months, and the results showed that 77% of patients had definite improvement. They noted that in the first month, 12% of patients were referred for surgical management, but none of the patients that showed a response to treatment in the first month required surgery. Lees and Turner[18] conducted another early study in 1963. They followed 51 patients with cervical spondylosis and radicular symptoms without myelopathy for 10 to 19 years. Some patients were exposed to conservative treatments, including wearing a cervical collar and manipulation, whereas others did not receive any treatment. At the end of the 10 years, 73% of patients reported having mild or no symptoms. DePlama and Subin[19] found significantly different results in 384 patients with cervical radiculopathy. This study compared surgical to nonsurgical outcomes and found that only 29% of conservatively treated patients attained complete symptom relief. Gore and colleagues[20] followed a group of 205 patients with neck pain, of whom 58% had radicular symptoms. Most of the patients were exposed to one or more treatments, including hospitalization, cervical collar, and oral medications. At the completion of the 10-year follow-up, 43% were pain-free and 79% reported a reduction in symptoms. However, 32% reported persistent moderate to severe pain. Two additional studies from the physiatry literature suggest that 70% to 90% of patients with cervical radiculopathy have a good outcome. However, each of these studies included some type of conservative management, including traction.[21,22] A more recent study of 563 patients who presented to the Mayo Clinic from 1976 to 1990 also showed that 90% of patients had mild or no symptoms after 4 to 5 years of follow-up. However, one-fifth of patients did not improve and ultimately underwent surgical treatment.[5] Only one study specifically monitored for recurrent symptoms and found that recurrences occurred in 12.5% of patients during a follow-up period of 1 to 2 years.[22]

Evolution of Radiographic Findings

The advent of computed tomography (CT) and magnetic resonance imaging (MRI) has significantly impacted the ability to diagnose and monitor disc herniations in patients with radiculopathy. These imaging studies have also made it possible to follow the natural course of disc herniations and compare the morphologic changes with symptomatic improvement. Key was the first to document the spontaneous regression of a herniated disc in the lumbar spine by myelography in 1945.[23] This phenomenon was confirmed with the use of follow-up CT scans in the lumbar and cervical spine in 1985.[24] Saal and colleagues[25] published a subsequent study in 1990 of 12 patients with documented lumbar herniations on CT. These patients were rescanned at an average of 25 months and the following findings were documented: 46% of subjects had 75% to 100% resorption, 36% had 50% to 75% decrease in herniation size, and 11% had 0% to 50% regression. They found that complete resorption was most frequently seen in the patients who had the largest herniations. However, they did not find a significant correlation between clinical and morphologic improvement. Bozzo and colleagues[26] had similar results regarding morphology of lumbar herniations on MRI: 48% of patients had greater than 70% reduction in size, 15% had a 30% to 50% reduction in size, 29% had no change, and 8% had an increase in size. Overall, 64% of the 69 patients had a reduction in herniation size, and the largest degree of resorption was seen in those with medium and large herniations. Maigne and Deligne[27] established a similar relationship between greater spontaneous resolutions in larger herniations in the cervical spine. Cowan and colleagues[28] performed repeat CT scans on 106 patients one year after being diagnosed with lumbosacral radiculopathy. Disc herniations that decreased or fully resolved were seen in 76% of patients. However, only 26% of disc bulges decreased or resolved. Masui and colleagues[29] found that disc herniation size decreased by 95% in 21 patients who had follow-up MRI imaging 7 to 10 years after being diagnosed with disc herniation and radiculopathy. Cribb and colleagues[30] focused on massive lumbar disc extrusions that obscured greater than 66% of the spinal canal at the time of diagnosis of radiculopathy. They found that after 25 months, 14 out of 15 herniations had completely resolved. Although Komori and colleagues[31] did not find a correlation between clinical symptom and radiological improvement, this finding has been demonstrated in more recent studies.[32] Dellerud and Nakstad[32] followed 92 patients over 14 months with follow-up CT scans and found a strong association between clinical improvement and reduction in the size of the lumbar herniation. They also found that central herniations and disc bulges were less likely to resolve, and the reduction in size of disc bulges was associated with a lesser degree of symptomatic improvement than with disc herniations.

SUMMARY

Radicular pain is a frequent complaint of patients presenting to outpatient primary care and musculoskeletal clinics. Based on a review of the literature, most cases of radiculopathy seem to be self-limiting and symptoms seem to resolve over the course of weeks to months. Advanced imaging has demonstrated the spontaneous resolution of disc herniations, particularly in larger protrusions and extrusions, and clinical improvement seems to correlate with morphologic resolution. Knowledge of the natural history of radiculopathy is crucial for the health care provider to appropriately counsel and treat patients with this disorder. Although each patient should be managed individually, the favorable prognosis of radiculopathy based on the natural history supports a conservative approach for the initial weeks to months for most patients.

REFERENCES

1. Deyo R, Weinstein J. Low back pain. N Engl J Med 2001;344(5):363–70.
2. Mixter W, Barr J. Rupture of the intervertebral disc with involvement of the spinal canal. N Engl J Med 1934;211:210–5.
3. Savettieri G, Salemi G, Rocca WA, et al. Prevalence of lumbosacral radiculopathy in two Sicilian municipalities. Acta Neurol Scand 1996;93(6):464–9.
4. Salemi G, Savettieri G, Meneghini F, et al. Prevalence of cervical spondylotic radiculopathy: a door-to-door survey in a Sicilian municipality. Acta Neurol Scand 1996;93:184–8.
5. Radhakrishan K, Litchy WJ, O'Fallon WM, et al. Epidemiology of cervical radiculopathy: a population-based study from Rochester, Minnesota, 1976 through 1990. Brain 1994;117:325–35.
6. Frymoyer JW. Back pain and sciatica. N Engl J Med 1988;318:291–300.
7. Weber H. Lumbar disc herniation. A controlled prospective study with ten years of observation. Spine 1983;8:131–40.
8. Heliovarra M, Makela M, Knekt P, et al. Determinants of sciatica and low back pain. Spine 1991;16:608–14.
9. Heikkila JK, Koskenvuo M, Heliovaara M, et al. Genetic and environmental factors in sciatica. Evidence from a nationwide panel of 9365 adult twin pairs. Ann Med 1989;21:393–8.
10. Varlotta GP, Brown MD, Kelsey JL, et al. Familial predisposition for herniation of a lumbar disc in patients who are less than twenty one years old. J Bone Joint Surg Am 1991;73:124–8.
11. Riihimaki H, Viikari-Juntura E, Moneta G, et al. Incidence of sciatic pain among men in machine operating, dynamic physical work and sedentary work. Spine 1994;19:138–42.
12. Miranda H, Viikari-Juntura E, Martikainen R, et al. Individual factors, occupational loading and physical exercise as predictors of sciatica pain. Spine 2002;27:1002–9.
13. Kelsey JL, Githens PB, O'Connor T, et al. Acute prolapsed lumbar intervertebral disc: an epidemiologic study with special reference to driving automobiles and cigarette smoking. Spine 1984;9:608–13.
14. Hakelius A. Prognosis in sciatica: a clinical follow-up of surgical and non surgical treatment. Acta Orthop Scand Suppl 1970;129:1–76.

15. Saal JA, Saal JS. Nonoperative treatment of herniated lumbar intervertebral disc with radiculopathy. Spine 1989;14(4):431–7.
16. Weber H, Holme I, Amilie E. The natural course of acute sciatica, with nerve root symptoms in a double blind placebo-controlled trial evaluating the effect of piroxicam. Spine 1993;18:1433–8.
17. Spurling R, Segerberg L. Lateral intervertebral disk lesions in the lower cervical region. JAMA 1953;151(5):354–9.
18. Lees F, Turner JW. Natural history and prognosis of cervical spondylosis. Br Med J 1963;2:1607–10.
19. DePalma, Sabin. Study of the cervical syndrome. Clin Orthop Relat Res 1965;32: 135–42.
20. Gore DR, Sepic SB, Gardner GM, et al. Neck pain: a long-term follow-up of 205 patients. Spine 1987;12(1):1–5.
21. Martin G, Corbin K. An evaluation of conservative treatment for patients with cervical disk syndrome. Arch Phys Med Rehabil 1954;35:87.
22. Honet J, Puri K. Cervical radiculitis: treatment and results in 82 patients. Arch Phys Med Rehabil 1976;57:12.
23. Key JA. The conservative and operative treatment of lesions of the intervertebral discs in the low back. Surgery 1945;17:291–303.
24. Teplick JG, Haskin ME. Spontaneous regression of herniated nucleus pulposus. AJR Am J Roentgenol 1985;145(2):371–5.
25. Saal JA, Saal JS, Herzog RJ. The natural history of lumbar intervertebral discs extrusions treated non-operatively. Spine 1990;20:1821–927.
26. Bozzao A, Gallucci M, Masciocchi C, et al. Lumbar disc herniation: MR imaging assessment of natural history in patients treated without surgery. Radiology 1992; 185:135–41.
27. Maigne JY, Deligne L. Computed tomographic follow-up study of 21 cases of nonoperatively treated cervical soft disc herniation. Spine 1994;19(2):189–91.
28. Cowan N, Bush K, Katz D, et al. The natural history of sciatica: a prospective radiological study. Clin Radiol 1992;46(2):7–12.
29. Masui T, Yukawa Y, Nakamura S, et al. Natural history of patients with lumbar disc herniation observed by magnetic resonance imaging for minimum 7 years. J Spinal Disord Tech 2005;18(2):121–6.
30. Cribb GL, Jaffray DC, Cassar-Pullicino VN. Observations on the natural history of massive lumbar disc herniation. J Bone Joint Surg Br 2007;89(6):782–4.
31. Komori H, Shinomiya K, Nakai O, et al. The natural history of herniated nucleus pulposus with radiculopathy. Spine 1996;21:225–9.
32. Dullerud R, Nakstad PH. CT changes after conservative treatment for lumbar disk herniation. Acta Radiol 1994;35(5):415–9.

Physical Examination in Radiculopathy

Arthur J. De Luigi, DO[a,b,c,*], Kevin F. Fitzpatrick, MD[a,b,d]

KEYWORDS

- Physical examination • Radiculopathy • Lumbar • Cervical

History and physical examination is the cornerstone in any clinician's foundation of knowledge in the appropriate diagnosis and treatment of any patient. To develop the best differential diagnosis, one must be aware of correlative signs and symptoms. A comprehensive physical examination is necessary to aid in determining distributions of symptoms and to lead one to the site of pathology. The focus of this article is on aiding the clinician in distinguishing radiculopathy from other causes of neck and low back pain.

DERMATOMES AND MYOTOMES

The term "dermatome" derives from the Greek roots *derma*, meaning skin, and *tome*, meaning segment. It is used to define a segment of skin whose sensory innervation is derived from a single spinal segment, spinal nerve, or nerve root. In the diagnosis of a radiculopathy, there is significant clinical utility in understanding the structures in the nervous system responsible for observed sensory deficits over a given area of skin. For example, if a segment of skin with sensory deficits can be reliably mapped to a single spinal nerve, this knowledge can be used to guide targeted therapy to that spinal nerve.

Since the late nineteenth century, efforts have been made to produce dermatomal maps, or visual representations of the various dermatomes.[1] Unfortunately, there has been a lack of consensus with regard to the precise localization of specific dermatomes. There are a variety of reasons why dermatomal mapping is difficult, and these have contributed to variable representations or maps. Four reasons are discussed.

The authors have nothing to disclose.

[a] Uniformed Services University of Health Sciences, Department of Neurology, 4301 Jones Bridge Road, Bethesda, MD 20814, USA
[b] Physical Medicine and Rehabilitation Residency, Walter Reed Army Medical Center, 6900 Georgia Avenue NW, Washington, DC 20307, USA
[c] Physical Medicine and Rehabilitation Service, Department of Orthopaedics and Rehabilitation, Walter Reed Army Medical Center, 6900 Georgia Avenue NW, Washington, DC 20307, USA
[d] Electrodiagnostic Medicine, Department of Orthopaedics and Rehabilitation, Walter Reed Army Medical Center, 6900 Georgia Avenue NW, Washington, DC 20307, USA
* Corresponding author. Physical Medicine and Rehabilitation Residency, Walter Reed Army Medical Center, 6900 Georgia Avenue NW, Washington, DC 20307.
E-mail address: arthur.deluigi@us.army.mil

Phys Med Rehabil Clin N Am 22 (2011) 7–40
doi:10.1016/j.pmr.2010.10.003
1047-9651/11/$ – see front matter. Published by Elsevier Inc.

1. Different anatomic structures can be expected to produce different maps. Although a segment of spinal cord is known to contribute many or most of its fibers to a single root and single spinal nerve, connections between roots exist.[2] Therefore, a sensory nerve fiber in the C5 spinal segment may not necessarily contribute to the C5 spinal nerve. As was stated by one author, "to view the spinal cord as composed of a series of independent spinal segments or neuromeres is convenient, but not accurate.[2]" As a result, differences can be expected to exist in the maps derived from spinal segments as compared with those derived from spinal nerves, which may account for some variability in dermatomal maps derived from various experimental techniques.

2. Multiple sensory modalities contribute to sensation in a particular segment of skin. Sensation to varying modalities is transmitted by varying nerve fibers. As a result, nerve fibers transmitting sensation to different modalities in the same area of skin may derive from different spinal nerves or different spinal segments. For example, a given area of skin may derive pain and temperature sensation from the C6 spinal nerve, but light touch sensation from the C7 spinal nerve; this can lead to confusion and disagreement among different representations of the dermatomal map.

3. Significant overlap exists between dermatomes. A given area of skin may receive sensation from more than one spinal nerve or spinal segment, which can explain the finding that even complete resection of a single spinal nerve may produce no loss of sensibility.[2,3] Because of the significant overlap between dermatomes, the classic drawing of a human body with distinct areas of skin representing the sensory domain of a particular neural element separated by well-defined lines is likely to be an oversimplification.

4. Significant challenges limit experimental procedures for defining dermatomes. Many techniques have been used to derive dermatomal maps. However, there are limitations to what can be performed experimentally. For example, it would be ethically questionable to experimentally sever human spinal nerves for the purpose of defining the resulting loss of sensation. Several techniques that have been used are described by Greenberg.[1] Among the techniques described are mapping areas of sensory loss in patients with known spinal or peripheral nerve injuries, documenting the locations of rashes in patients with herpes zoster, experimental sectioning of nerve roots in animals, defining areas of sensory loss with surgically confirmed radiculopathy due to disc herniation, and one investigator went so far as to section his own superficial radial nerve to describe the resulting area of sensory loss. None of these experimental techniques is without flaw, and the varying ways in which dermatomal maps have been studied may explain some of their differences.

Similar to a dermatome, the term myotome is used to describe all of the muscles that receive innervation from a single spinal segment or spinal nerve. Significant overlap in myotomes occurs in a similar fashion to dermatomes. Nearly every muscle receives motor nerve fibers from more than one spinal level. Although many muscles have a dominant innervating nerve root, to consider a muscle to be innervated by a single spinal level is not accurate. For many of the same reasons cited above explaining the difficulty in constructing dermatomal maps, there is some disagreement and overlap among varying sources with regard to the spinal levels responsible for the innervation of particular muscles.

With the availability of electrodiagnostic testing, it is possible to study myotomal distributions in human subjects. By performing electrodiagnostic testing on subjects with confirmed single spinal nerve lesions, studies have been designed to determine which muscles receive innervation from a given spinal nerve. Similarly, a single spinal nerve can be electrically stimulated at the time of spinal surgery, and observation of the muscles in which contraction subsequently occurs can be used to define myotomal distributions. Corollaries to mapping dermatomal distributions using similar sensory techniques are not readily available. Several attempts have been made to define myotomal distributions using these techniques.[4–8]

Despite the seemingly straightforward design of these studies, differences in results can be found. For example, Brendler[5] found that on electrical stimulation of the C6 nerve root, contraction of the flexor carpi radialis occurred in 0 of 3 patients tested. However, Levin and colleagues[6] found that in subjects with surgically confirmed single-level C6 radiculopathies, 4 out of 5 had electrodiagnostic abnormalities in the flexor carpi radialis. This discrepancy, along with others of a similar nature, leaves the reader to wonder about the true contribution of specific nerve roots to the innervation of individual muscles.

Despite these significant challenges, knowledge and understanding of the general concepts of dermatomal and myotomal distributions can be extremely valuable in the clinical evaluation of a suspected radiculopathy. Even if discrepancies exist, there is general agreement on the spinal nerves that provide innervation to most muscles. Similarly, general agreement exists with regard to the approximate sensory distribution of each spinal nerve. When a patient presents with a suspected radiculopathy, a detailed neurologic examination should be performed to include manual muscle testing to determine the distribution of weakness as well as sensory testing to determine the distribution of impaired sensation. If there is correlation in the suspected root levels responsible for sensation in the impaired distribution with those contributing innervation to the muscles found to be weak, this may lead to a diagnosis of involvement of a particular root level based on the physical examination.

Caution must be applied in using physical examination findings to exclude a radiculopathy. Lauder and colleagues[9] showed that in subjects with electrodiagnostic evidence of a radiculopathy, as many as 31% will have no weakness on physical examination and as many as 45% will have no sensory abnormalities detected on physical examination. Based on these results, it is likely that a significant proportion of patients who present with a true radiculopathy may have a normal physical examination.

There are several reasons that a patient with a radiculopathy may have normal physical examination findings. As discussed, the significant overlap between dermatomes results in each segment of skin receiving sensory innervation from more than one spinal nerve. Therefore if a single spinal nerve is injured, the other overlapping spinal nerves will continue to provide at least partial sensation to the area of skin in question. In fact, it would be unusual for a patient with a single-level radiculopathy to have gross loss of sensation.

Furthermore, weakness may not be present even in a severe radiculopathy. There are several reasons for this observation. First, a radiculopathy often involves injury to only a fraction of the fibers contained in the spinal nerve.[10] It would require degeneration or conduction block of a relatively large proportion of axons contributing innervation to a particular muscle before weakness were observed clinically. In addition, as already discussed, nearly all muscles receive innervation from more than one spinal nerve. Therefore, strength can be preserved if axons from other spinal nerves remain intact even in a very severe single-level radiculopathy.

When physical examination findings are present, they can be very helpful in diagnosing a radiculopathy and identifying the involved level. This identification requires an understanding of dermatomal and myotomal distributions. Despite challenges that are present in interpreting dermatomal and myotomal maps, they can be very useful in the evaluation of a radiculopathy (**Table 1**).

CERVICAL SPINE
Provocative Tests

There is a wide variety of provocative tests and signs described in the literature (**Table 2**) regarding physical examination of the cervical spine to evaluate radiculopathy. In addition to the variance in the nomenclature of these tests, there are multiple descriptions on how these tests should be properly performed. Review of the literature reveals multiple review articles evaluating physical examination for cervical radiculopathy,[11–27] as well as a volume of evidence-based studies evaluating the validity and reliability of the tests; however, for other tests there is limited or no existing scientific literature.

Spurling test (foraminal compression test, neck compression test, quadrant test)

During World War II, while working at the Walter Reed General Hospital, Roy Greenwood Spurling, the hospital's first Chief of Neurosurgery and organizer of neurosurgery for the entire Army, first noted this finding in patients with ruptured cervical discs. During this time, Spurling and Scoville[28] had demonstrated a positive test on 12 patients with presumed ruptured cervical discs who were confirmed surgically in 1943, and reported their findings in 1944. The original description of the test by Spurling and Scoville[28] explained that the head and neck will be tilted toward the painful side to reproduce the patient's typical radicular symptoms. Pressure will then be placed on the top of the head to further intensify the symptoms, whereas tilting the head away from the painful side will alleviate the symptoms. At present the test, also known as the foraminal compression test, neck compression test, or the quadrant test, is performed by neck extension, rotation, and downward pressure on the head with a positive finding eliciting radicular pain into the ipsilateral arm of head rotation.[23] Overall, the Spurling test has been described as "almost pathognomonic of a cervical intraspinal lesion."[19,28]

Recent reviewers in the past several years who completed evaluating the validity of the various cervical provocative maneuvers including the Spurling test concluded that the test demonstrated low to moderate sensitivity and high specificity,[13,14,18] and a good interrater reliability.[18] A study by Shah and Rajshekhar[29] in 2004 evaluated the test on 50 surgical patients with findings on magnetic resonance imaging (MRI). The results of the study were that the Spurling test was 92% sensitive and 95% specific, with a positive predictive value of 96.4% and a negative predictive value of 90.9%, concluding that the Spurling test is the gold standard for evaluating cervical radiculopathy.[29] Additional studies on the reliability[30] and validity[31] revealed that interrater reliability for the Spurling test in a seated position had a kappa coefficient of 0.40 to 0.77, and a sensitivity of 40% to 60% and specificity of 92% to 100%. Their conclusions were that the Spurling test had good interrater reliability when testing with the patient in a seated position, and that the test has a high specificity but low sensitivity.[30,31]

When evaluating the correlation of a positive Spurling test with findings on electrodiagnostics, the Spurling test had a (6/20) sensitivity of 30% and a specificity of (160/172) 93%.[32] There were 2 other studies[33,34] that did not use the most widely accepted description of a positive Spurling test or used spinal cord deformity as the criterion, and therefore, their contribution to evidence-based evaluation of the Spurling test is limited.

Overall, the recent contributions to the literature have lent significance toward the utility of the Spurling test in the physical examination of patients with suspected cervical radiculopathy.

Lhermitte sign
The Lhermitte sign, also known as the Barber Chair phenomenon, is named after Jacques Jean Lhermitte,[35–37] who described findings in 1920 when evaluating patients with spinal cord concussion and later in other neurologic diagnoses. However, the sign was previously described by both Marie and Chatelin[38] in 1917 and Babinski and Dubois[39] in 1918. While evaluating patients with head injuries, Marie and Chatelin[38] noted transient pins and needles sensations into the limbs on flexion of the neck. Babinski and Dubois[39] noted electric discharges into the limbs with head flexion, sneezing, or coughing in a patient with Brown-Sequard syndrome.

There are still variations of how the Lhermitte sign is described; however, current description of positive findings is elicited by flexion of the neck producing electric shock-like sensations that extend down the spine and shoot into the limbs. The findings have been described in various pathologic states caused by trauma to the cervical portion of the spinal cord, multiple sclerosis, cervical cord tumor, cervical spondylosis, or even vitamin B12 deficiency.[23–25]

There is limited literature evaluating the effectiveness of the Lhermitte sign in determining cervical radiculopathy. A review by Malanga and colleagues[18] concluded that there is insufficient evidence of the interrater reliability, sensitivity, and specificity of the Lhermitte sign specifically. However, the active flexion and extension test described by Sandmark and Nissell[33] resembles the Lhermitte sign, and was found to have a high specificity (90%) and low sensitivity (27%) with a negative predictive value of 75% and positive predictive value of 55%. Another study reviewed the Lhermitte test in assessing cervical cord lesions, and reported a high sensitivity and low specificity.[34]

Based on the lack of any recent or previous evidence literature regarding the validity or reliability of the Lhermitte sign, its usefulness in the examination of cervical radiculopathy is limited.

Shoulder abduction test (shoulder abduction relief sign)
In addition to the contribution of the Spurling test, Spurling also was the first to report the shoulder abduction relief sign, more commonly known as the shoulder abduction test, in 1956. The initial description was the relief of radicular symptoms by raising the arm above the head.[40] The shoulder abduction test is now currently described as active or passive abduction of the ipsilateral shoulder. The hand rests on the top of the head, and a positive test is elicited with the relief or reduction of ipsilateral cervical radicular symptoms.[41]

There is limited evidence regarding the validity and reliability of the shoulder abduction test. Both studies in the literature were conducted by Viikari-Juntura and colleagues,[30,31] and revealed fair interrater reliability (kappa 0.21–0.40),[30] proportion of specific agreement (0.57–0.67), with high specificity (80%–100%) and low sensitivity (43%–50%).[31] However, a review by Malanga and colleagues[18] concluded that the test had good interrater reliability with high specificity and low sensitivity.

There are several studies evaluating the effectiveness in diagnosing radicular pain from shoulder pain[25] as well as disc pathology versus spondylosis[42]; however, the evidence is limited.

The shoulder abduction test has been claimed to be predictive of excellent response to surgical treatment. The shoulder abduction test had positive relief in

Table 1
Dermatomes and myotomes

Muscle	Primary Root(s) from Brendler[5]	Other Root(s) from Brendler[5]	Negative Root(s) from Brendler[5] (Roots not Contributing)	Primary Root(s) from Levin[6]	Other Root(s) from Levin[6]
Flexor carpi ulnaris	C7, C8		C6		
Extensor digitorum communis	C8	C7		C7, C8	C6
Extensor carpi ulnaris	C8	C7			
Abductor pollicis longus	C8		C7		
Extensor pollicis longus	C8		C7		
Teres minor	C6	C7, C8			
Teres major	C6	C7, C8			
Latissimus dorsi	C6	C7, C8			
Triceps	C7, C8	C6		C7	C6, C8
Brachioradialis	C5		C6	C5,6	
Flexor carpi radialis	C7		C6	C6, C7	
Abductor pollicis brevis	C8			C8	
Extensor carpi radialis	C6	C5, C7	C8	C6, C7	
Pronator teres	C6	C7			
Flexor digitorum Profundus	C8		C7		
Pronator quadratus	C6	C7		C8	
Flexor pollicis longus	C8		C7		
Deltoid	C5	C3, C4, C6, C7		C5	C6
Biceps	C5, C6	C7		C5,6	
Pectoralis major	C7, C8	C6	C5		
Levator scapula	C3	C4	C5		
Trapezius	C1, C2, C3, C4				
Supraspinatus				C5,6	

	Primary Root(s) from Tsao[7]	Other Root(s) from Tsao[7]	Primary Root(s) from Phillips[8]	Other Root(s) from Phillips[8]
Infraspinatus			C5	
Anconeus			C7, 8	C6
Extensor indicis proprius			C8	C7
First dorsal interosseus			C8	C7
Abductor digiti minimi			C8	
Adductor longus	L2, L3, L4		L3	L2, L4
Iliacus	L2, L3, L4		L3	L2, L4
Vastus lateralis	L2, L4		L3	L2, L4
Rectus femoris	L4			
Vastus medialis	L3, L4			
Posterior tibialis	L5	S1		
Tibialis anterior	L5		L4, L5	S1
Extensor digitorum brevis	L5			
Peroneus longus	L5		L5	S1, L4
Extensor hallucis longus	L5	S1		
Gluteus medius	L5	S1		
Semitendinosus	L5			
Tensor fascia lata	L5			
Medial gastrocnemius	S1	L5	S1	L5, S2
Lateral gastrocnemius	S1	L5	S1	L5, S2
Abductor digiti quinti pedis	S1			
Biceps femoris short head	S1			
Biceps femoris long head	S1			
Gluteus maximus	S1	L5	S1	L5, S2
Abductor hallucis	S1	L5		

Table 2
Provocative maneuvers for the evaluation of cervical and lumbar radiculopathy

	Design	Number	Measures	Lumbar Control	Results	Conclusion
Ekedahl et al,[106] 2010	Cross-sectional validity study	75	Roland Morris Disability Questionnaire (RMDQ), SLR, Fingertip to floor test, Slump	Slump test	RMDQ/FTF (0.68 men, 0.70 women); RMDQ/SLR (0.60 women, 0.28 men)	Good validity of FTF with both sexes, but SLR has less value especially for men
Suri et al,[59] 2010	Cross-sectional with prospective recruitment		FST, CFST, medial ankle pinprick sensation, sit to stand, patellar reflex, Achilles reflex, anterior thigh sensation, hip abductor strength	None	Midlumbar impingement: FST, CFST, medial ankle pinprick sensation, and patellar reflex testing demonstrated LRs ≥5.0 (LR infinity). LRs ≥5.0 observed with combinations of FST and either patellar reflex testing (LR 7.0; 95% confidence interval [CI] 2.3–21) or the sit-to-stand test (LR infinity). Low lumbar impingement: Achilles reflex test demonstrated an LR ≥5.0 (LR 7.1; 95% CI 0.96–53); test combinations did not increase LRs. Level-specific impingement: LRs ≥5.0 were observed	Individual tests alter likelihood of mid, low lumbar, and level-specific impingement; test combinations improve diagnostic accuracy for midlumbar impingement

					for anterior thigh sensation at L2 (LR 13; 95% CI 1.8–87); FST at L3 (LR 5.7; 95% CI 2.3–4.4); patellar reflex testing (LR 7.7; 95% CI 1.7–35), medial ankle sensation (LR infinity), or CFST (LR 13; 95% CI 1.8–87) at L4; and hip abductor strength at L5 (LR 11; 95% CI 1.3–84). Test combinations increased LRs for level-specific root impingement at the L4 level only	
Barz et al,[132] 2010	Retrospective case studies	200	Nerve root sedimentation sign (radiologic)	Nonspecific LBP (no leg pain, claudication, dural sac CSA >120 mm, walk >1 km) versus symptomatic LSS (+leg pain, claudication, CSA <80 mm, walk <200 m)	Positive sedimentation sign identified in 94 patients in the LSS group (94%; 95% CI, 90%–99%) but none in the LBP group (0%; 95% CI, 0%–4%). Reliability was kappa = 1.0 (intraobserver) and kappa = 0.93 (interobserver), respectively. No difference in the detection between segmental levels L1–L5 in the LSS group	Positive sedimentation exclusive and reliable, suggesting high specificity and sensitivity

(continued on next page)

Table 2
(continued)

	Design	Number	Lumbar		Results	Conclusion
			Measures	Control		
van der Windt et al,[60] 2010	Cochrane review	16 cohort and 3 case-control	Scoliosis, paresis or muscle weakness, muscle wasting, impaired reflexes, sensory deficits, forward flexion, hyperextension test, slump test, SLR, CSLR	Back pain with diagnostic imaging or findings at surgery	Scoliosis, paresis or muscle weakness, muscle wasting, impaired reflexes, sensory deficits were poor; forward flexion, hyperextension test, and slump test performed slightly better; SLR (surgical) high prevalence of disc herniation (58%–98%) showed high sensitivity (pooled estimate 0.92, 95% CI: 0.87 to 0.95) with widely varying specificity (0.10–1.00, pooled estimate 0.28, 95% CI: 0.18–0.40); CSLR showed high specificity (pooled estimate 0.90, 95% CI: 0.85–0.94) with consistently low sensitivity (pooled estimate 0.28, 95% CI: 0.22–0.35). Combining positive test results increased the specificity of physical tests, but few studies presented data on test combinations	Poor diagnostic performance of most physical tests; however, most from surgical populations and may not apply to primary care or nonselected populations. Better performance may be obtained when tests are combined

Coster et al,[61] 2010	Prospective	202	SLR, history, EMG	Radiologic nerve root compression (95 patients)	Dermatomal radiation (odds ratio [OR] 2.1), more pain on coughing, sneezing, or straining (OR 2.4), positive straight leg raising (OR 3.0), and ongoing denervation on EMG (OR 4.5)	History and physical helpful in predicting nerve root compression on MRI; EMG may have additional value
Summers et al,[118] 2009	Diagnostic validity	67	Flip test, SLR	Supine straight leg raise	33% no pain, 39% pain on full knee extension, 28% resisted extension due to pain	All patients had +Flip compared with supine SLR below 45°
Last and Hulbert,[62] 2009	Review					Focus on tx, not dx
Rubenstein et al,[13] 2008	Review		SLR	Other neurologic signs and tests	SLR consistently reported sensitive for radicular pain, but limited by low specificity	SLR high sensitivity, low specificity
Majlesi et al,[82] 2008	Prospective case control	75	Slump, SLR, Lasegue	Absence or presence of disc herniation on MRI	Slump test more sensitive (0.84) than the SLR (0.52) with lumbar disc herniations. However, SLR slightly more specific test (0.89) than the slump test (0.83)	Slump test higher sensitivity, SLR more specific
Freynhagen et al,[133] 2008	Prospective	43	Sensory testing: vibration, hair contact, cold	Pseudoradicular, healthy normals, radicular pain	Vibration detection was the most sensitive parameter with 73% abnormal values in radicular and 47% in pseudoradicular cases	Vibration testing

(continued on next page)

Table 2
(continued)

	Design	Number	Measures	Lumbar Control	Results	Conclusion
Chou et al,[63] 2007	Review					Guide toward imaging and treatment
Rabin et al,[105] 2007	Cohort	71	Seated versus Supine SLR	MRI findings	Supine SLR test sensitivity 67% compared with seated SLR sensitivity 41%	Supine SLR higher sensitivity
Miller,[64] 2007	Descriptive					Focus on how to perform, not evidence based
van Rijn et al,[65] 2006	Prospective	75	VAS during examination	MRI findings	MRI abnormal 74% symptomatic, 33% asymptomatic	Two-thirds of patients poor predicative value
Nadler et al,[107] 2004	Retrospective	200	SLR, strength, sensation, reflexes	Personal injury, workman's compensation	Positive SLR in women 7.4 more likely in PIP versus WC (95% CI, 11.1–992.6; $P<.001$). Men, bilateral SLR was 38.9 times more likely PIP (95% CI, 11.3–133.6; $P<.001$)	Higher rates of positive SLR in PIP versus WC

Study	Type	N	Tests	Imaging	Results	Comments
Vroomen et al,[66] 2002	Prospective	274	Paresis, tendon reflexes, +SLR, and finger to floor	MRI findings	SLR not predictive, independent diagnostic value of paresis and finger to floor distance	Tests generally have lower sensitivity and specificity than previously reported
Nadler et al,[127] 2001	Case study	2	FNST, crossed FNST	FNST	Upper lumbar radiculopathy confirmed by FNST and crossed FNST	May be a valuable screening tool
Patel and Ogle,[67] 2000	Review					Focus on tx, not dx
Deville et al,[95] 2000	Review		SLR		Overall, pooled data SLR: sensitivity 91%, specificity 26%. CSLR: sensitivity 29%, specificity 88%	SLR: high sensitivity and low specificity; CSLR: high specificity, low sensitivity
Manifold and McCann,[22] 1999	Review					H&P can lead to appropriate imaging and EMG
Humphreys,[68] 1999	Review					Focus on tx, not dx
Stankovic et al,[116] 1999			Slump, Braggard		94% positive slump with frank disc herniation, 78% bulging discs, 75% without disc finding	High prevalence of findings in patients without pathology

(continued on next page)

Table 2
(continued)

	Design	Number	Measures	Lumbar Control	Results	Conclusion
Supik and Broom,[103] 1994			Bowstring sign		71 % positive sign in patients with known lumbar disc herniation	
Alexander et al,[119] 1992	Retrospective	154	Negative extension sign (ability to achieve full extension), SLR, CSLR	EMG, CT, myelography, DTR, sensory and motor deficits	By day 5 94 able to fully extend, 19 of 33 patients with + extension sign on admission became negative within 5 days of admission: 95% satisfaction, 90% without job changes	Extension sign effectively predicts a favorable response to nonoperative therapy of HNP in 91% of cases
Kosteljanetz et al,[81] 1988	Prospective	100	SLR (leg pain, leg or back pain)		Leg pain: sensitivity 76%, specificity 45%, prevalence 58%; Leg or back pain: sensitivity 91%, specificity 21%, prevalence 58%	Adding back pain will increase sensitivity but decrease specificity

Hong et al,[26] 1986	Retrospective	108		Clinical findings correlate with EMG findings to greater extent than radiographic findings	EMG beneficial to provide accurate assessment
Kosteljanetz et al,[86] 1984	Prospective	52	SLR (leg pain, leg or back pain)	SLR: (leg pain) sensitivity 89%, specificity 17%, prevalence 86% (leg or back pain): sensitivity 95%, specificity 14%, prevalence 86%; CSLR: (contralateral leg pain) sensitivity 24%, specificity 96%, prevalence 86% (contralateral leg pain or back pain): sensitivity 42%, specificity 85%, prevalence 86%	Adding back pain will increase sensitivity but decrease specificity
Hudgins,[110] 1979	Prospective	274	CSLR	Sensitivity 24%, specificity 96%, prevalence 83%	

(continued on next page)

Table 2
(continued)

	Design	Number	Measures	Control	Results	Conclusion
Lumbar						
Spangfort,[83] 1972	Prospective	2504	Lasegue (SLR), CSLR		SLR: sensitivity 97% (73% from L1/L2–L3/4), specificity 11%, prevalence 88%; CSLR: sensitivity 23%, specificity 88%, prevalence 86%	SLR: high sensitivity and low specificity, decreased specificity for upper lumbar level; CSLR: high specificity, low sensitivity
Hakelius,[93] 1972	Prospective	1986	SLR, CSLR		Sensitivity 96%, specificity 15%, prevalence 75%	High sensitivity and low specificity
Charnley,[92] 1951	Prospective	88	SLR		Leg or back pain: sensitivity 91%, specificity 21%, prevalence 58%	Moderate sensitivity and specificity
Cervical						
	Design	Number	Measures	Control	Results	Conclusion
Eubanks,[11] 2010	Review					Focus on tx, not dx
Kuijper et al,[12] 2009	Review		Foraminal compression test	MRI, EMG	No well-defined criteria and not properly evaluated	Poor clinical predictive value
Rubenstein et al,[13] 2008	Review		Spurling, ULTT	Other neurologic signs and tests	Spurling high specificity, ULTT high sensitivity	Value with Spurling and upper limb tension test
Nordin et al,[15] 2008	Review	95 articles	Numerous test		Manual provocation test high predictive value	Validity of most tests are lacking
Guzman et al,[16] 2008	Review		4 grades		Focus on triage to 4 grades	Focus on guiding treatment

Study	Design	N	Tests	Reference standard	Results	Comments
Rubenstein et al,[14] 2007	Review	6 studies	Spurling, upper limb tension test, traction/distraction, Valsalva	Various reference standards	Spurling, traction/distraction, and Valsalva demonstrated low to moderate sensitivity and high specificity, ULTT high sensitivity and low specificity	Spurling, traction/distraction, Valsalva will rule in, and negative ULTT will rule out
Rainville et al,[134] 2007	Case series	55	MMT of forearm pronation versus WE, EF, EE	Diagnostic imaging evidence	C6 radiculopathies forearm pronation weakness 72% (twice as common as WE, present in all with EF/WE weakness, and all but 2 with EE weakness); C7 radiculopathies forearm pronation weakness only 10% of subjects	Forearm pronation weakness is the most frequent motor finding in C6 radiculopathies, and may be found in some cases of C7
Shah and Rajshekhar,[29] 2004	Prospective	50	Spurling	Surgical/MRI findings	Spurling 92% sensitive, 95% specific, PPV 96.4%, NPV 90.9%	Spurling is gold standard
Douglass and Bope,[20] 2004	Review					Focus on tx, not dx
Malanga et al,[18] 2003	Review		Spurling, shoulder abduction relief test, neck distraction test, Lhermitte, Hoffman, Adson		High specificity, low sensitivity with good interexaminer reliability: Spurling, neck distraction, and shoulder abduction relief test. Hoffman: no evidence of interexaminer reliability, fair sensitivity, fair to good specificity. Lhermitte/Adson: no existing literature on reliability, sensitivity, or specificity	Spurling, shoulder abduction, and neck distraction highest level of evidence in predicting radiculopathy

(continued on next page)

Table 2
(continued)

			Cervical		
	Design	Number	Measures	Control	Results	Conclusion
Wainner et al,[21] 2003	Prospective	82	Numerous test	EMG	Combination of tests better than any single test, however ULTT most useful for ruling out	Combination best to rule in, ULTT best to rule out
Tong et al,[32] 2002	Cross-sectional	255	Spurling	EMG	Spurling sensitivity of 6/20 (30%), specificity of 160/172 (93%). Positive in 16.6% normal group, 3.4% of group with nerve disorders other than radiculopathy, 25% of the group with abnormality not consistent with any specific diagnosis group, in 37.5% of group with possible radiculopathy, and 40% of the group with certain radiculopathy	Spurling low sensitivity, but is specific for radiculopathy diagnosed by EMG

Study	Design	N	Test	Comparison	Results	Conclusion
Sung and Wang,[55] 2001	Prospective	16	Hoffman's reflex + in asymptomatic patients	Asymptomatic patients MRI cervical pathology	14 spondylosis, 16 had MRI findings, 15 had cervical cord compression with HNP (other had T5–6 disc compression)	Presence of Hoffman in "asymptomatic" patients strongly suggest underlying pathology
Haig et al,[135] 1999	Prospective	252	Physical examination	EMG	EMG altered 42% of dx, confirmed 37%, and did not clarify 21%	Necessary to have examination with EMG for accurate diagnosis
Dvorak,[69] 1998	Review					Focus on advanced imaging and EMG
Malanga,[23] 1997	Review					Focus on detailed H&P to guide treatment and return to play
Sandmark,[33] 1995	Prospective, single-blind	75	Five manual tests: neck rotation, active flexion/extension, ULTT, palpation, foraminal test	None	Palpation good screening; foraminal and ULTT caused pain in almost all patients, but inconsistent radicular symptoms, neck rotation or flexion/extension insufficient sensitivity	Palpation initial screen, ULTT and foraminal testing may also help

(continued on next page)

Table 2
(continued)

	Design	Number	Cervical Measures	Control	Results	Conclusion
Ellenberg et al,[24] 1994	Review					Examination to guide advanced diagnostics
Viikari-Juntura,[31] 1989	Prospective	43	Spurling, shoulder abduction (relief) sign, neck distraction		Spurling: sensitivity 40%–60%, specificity 92%–100%; shoulder abduction relief sign: sensitivity 43%–50%, specificity 80%–100%; neck distraction: sensitivity 40%–43%, specificity 100%	Spurling, shoulder abduction relief, and neck distraction: high specificity, low sensitivity
Viikari-Juntura,[30] 1987	Prospective	52	Spurling, shoulder abduction (relief) sign, neck distraction		Spurling: kappa 0.40–0.77, PSA 0.47–0.80; shoulder abduction relief sign: kappa 0.21–0.40, PSA 0.57–0.67; neck distraction: kappa 0.50, PSA 0.71	Spurling: fair to excellent; shoulder abduction relief: fair; neck distraction: good reliability

Abbreviations: CFNT, crossed femoral nerve test; CFST, crossed femoral stress test; CSA, cross-sectional area; CSLR, crossed straight leg raise; DTR, deep tendon reflex; dx, diagnosis; EE, elbow extensor; EF, elbow flexor; EMG, electromyogram; FNST, femoral nerve stretch test; FST, femoral stress test; FTF, fingertip to floor; H&P, history and physicals; HNP, herniated nucleus pulposus; LBP, lower back pain; LR, likelihood ratio; LSS, lumbar spinal stenosis; MMT, manual muscle test; MRI, magnetic resonance imaging; NPV, negative predictive value; PIP, personal injury protection; PPV, positive predictive value; PSA, proportion of specific agreement; SLR, straight leg raise; tx, therapy; ULTT, upper limb tension test; VAS, visual analog scale; WC, workman's compensation; WE, wrist extensor.

15 of 22 patients who failed conservative management of cervical radicular symptoms, and confirmed disc pathology on myelography[40]; however, this study had a small sample size and did not provide significant outcome measures. The shoulder abduction relief maneuver has also been reported to benefit patients by incorporating it into a nonsurgical treatment plan.[43]

Overall, the review of the evidence-based literature reveals that currently there is limited research on the validity and reliability for the use of the shoulder adbuction test in the diagnosis of cervical radiculopathy.

Upper limb tension test

The upper limb tension test (ULTT), as described as brachial plexus tension test (BPTT) or test of Elvey, is a lesser known test used in the evaluation of cervical radiculopathy versus brachial plexus. The ULTT appears to offer a means of examining the extensibility and mechanosensitivity of the neural tissues related to an upper limb. It is performed in a sequence of movements with the patient supine. The following sequences of motions are performed: scapular depression, shoulder abduction, forearm supination, wrist and finger extension, shoulder lateral elevation, elbow extension, and contralateral/ipsilateral cervical side bending. The test is positive if one or more of the following occurs: radicular symptoms are reproduced, side-to-side difference in elbow extension is greater than 10°, contralateral cervical side bending increases symptoms, or ipsilateral side bending decreases symptoms.[13,14,21,33,44,45]

Wainner and colleagues[21] evaluated several provocative tests for the diagnosis of cervical radiculopathy, and concluded that the ULTT was the most useful test for ruling out cervical radiculopathy,[21] whereas Sandmark and Nisell,[33] in a study of 75 patients, concluded that the ULTT caused pain in almost all patients. The study by Quintner[44] revealed a high sensitivity (83%) and a low specificity (11%). The reviews by Rubenstein and colleagues[13,14] concluded that the ULTT demonstrated high sensitivity and low specificity.

Overall there is limited evidence regarding the utility of the ULTT in the diagnosis of cervical radiculopathy.

Neck distraction test (manual traction test)

Another infrequently described provocative test is the neck distraction test, also known as the manual traction test. The description on the proper performance of the test is for the examiner to place one hand on the occiput and the other on the chin while slowly lifting the patient. A positive finding is noted when the pain is diminished during the distraction.[41]

Two fairly recent reviews of various provocative tests were conducted that evaluated the current literature supporting the use of the neck distraction test to aid in the diagnosis of cervical radiculopathy. Malanga and colleagues[18] concluded that existing literature appears to indicate high specificity, low sensitivity, and good to fair interexaminer reliability for the neck distraction test,[18] whereas Rubenstein and colleagues[13,14] felt there was low to moderate sensitivity and high specificity.

In reviewing the literature, the lone studies to evaluate reliability and validity were conducted Viikari-Juntura's group[30,31] in 1987 and 1989. The findings in these studies demonstrated good reliability, with kappa values ranging from 0.50 to 0.71, and a high specificity (100%) and low sensitivity (40%–43%).

Overall, there is limited evidence regarding the neck distraction test in the assessment of cervical radicular symptoms.

Hoffmann sign

Historically there have been several variations of the Hoffman sign and controversy regarding its true clinical significance.[46–58] The Hoffman sign is commonly assessed in the evaluation of the cervical spine. Although it does not indicate cervical radiculopathy, it is useful in the physical examination in determination of the etiology of the symptoms. There are differences in the descriptions of the test and what constitutes a positive finding. The criteria in some studies have been lenient with a positive finding as flexion of the thumb, index finger, or both. On reexamination these positives were later stratified into "true" (flexion of both thumb and index finger) or "incomplete" (with flexion of either).[49]

There has been vast disagreement regarding the clinical significance and whether the phenomenon is pathologic or physiologic.[49,51,58] There have been several studies on the incidence of a positive response in normal patients or patients without any clear pathology, with an incidence of 1.63% to 3.4%.[49,51,53] However, the prevailing thought is that it is an upper motor neuron (UMN) sign indicating that there is pyramidal tract involvement.[49,51] If the Hoffman sign truly indicates a UMN disorder such as cervical myelopathy and cord compression, there is enormous value in separating cervical radiculopathy from the differential diagnosis.

There is no current literature evaluating the interrater reliability, and limited literature on the validity of the Hoffman test. The study by Raaf[58] evaluated 124 patients with cervical complaints and advance neuroimaging, and revealed a sensitivity of 58% and specificity of 78%, with a positive predictive value of 62% and negative predictive value of 75%.

Overall, there is no evidence specifically evaluating the Hoffman sign for radiculopathy; however, it may be beneficial in the determination of possible cord versus root injury.

PHYSICAL EXAMINATION OF LUMBAR RADICULOPATHY
Provocative Tests

In the review of the literature regarding physical examination of the lumbar spine to evaluate radiculopathy, there is a wide variety of provocative tests and signs (see **Table 2**). There is variance in both the nomenclature of these tests as well as their descriptions. There are numerous reviews evaluating the various tests.[13,59–70] For some of these tests there has been a volume of evidence collected regarding their validity and reliability; however, for some of the less commonly discussed tests there is limited to no existing literature.

Straight leg raise/Lasegue sign/Lazarevič sign

The straight leg raise (SLR) test is commonly used to test the provocation of radicular symptoms for lumbar pathology. The SLR has been described in the literature since the late nineteenth century by numerous investigators, and subsequent eponyms have described the slight variations in testing.

The first documented description of the SLR was described in 1880 by the Serbian neurologist Laza K. Lazarevič[70] in the Serbian Archives in 6 patients said to have increased pain while stretching the sciatic nerve. Lazarevič[71] then fully described the sign in 1884 with a multiple-step approach; the classic SLR test is the third step, in which the supine patient raises the leg with an extended knee until he or she begins to feel pain, at which point the angle of elevation is documented.

The more commonly referenced Lasegue sign was initially described in 1881 by J.J. Frost, a pupil of the French internist Ernest-Charles Lasegue. Frost[72] described that pain could be elicited in the distribution of the sciatic nerve during leg elevation while maintaining pressure on the knee to promote extension. He believed that pressure from the hamstring on the nerve is the mechanism for pain. An alternative mechanism of pathology was postulated by Lucien de Beurmann in 1884. His conclusion was that the sciatic nerve was being stretched during leg elevation rather than from muscle compression.[73] There have been several studies[74–77] to support this pathophysiologic stress by measuring distal downward migration of the spinal nerve ranging from 2 to 7 mm.

Through the historical references and descriptions, the consensus positive finding using the classic SLR test is the elicitation of radicular pain down the posterior thigh below the knee with the patient supine and the leg with knee extended being raised between 30° and 70°.[78] Pain below 30° or beyond 70° is unlikely to be from nerve root irritation and more likely to be secondary to tight gluteal or hamstring musculature.[79–81]

The SLR test has been used as the primary test to diagnose lumbar disc herniations and has been found to have high correlation with findings on operation, because its sensitivity is high in only disc herniations leading to root compression that may eventually need operation.[82] A review of the current literature evaluating the validity of the SLR test reveals numerous studies evaluating the prevalence, sensitivity, and specificity of the SLR test. The majority of these studies focus on surgical confirmation of the preoperative findings on physical examination. A recent Cochrane review evaluating physical examination for lumbar radiculopathy due to disc herniation[60] included 16 cohort studies and 3 case-control series. Most studies assessed the SLR test. In surgical populations, characterized by a high prevalence of disc herniation (58%–98%), the SLR test showed high sensitivity (pooled estimate 0.92, 95% confidence interval [CI]: 0.87–0.95) with widely varying specificity (0.10–1.00, pooled estimate 0.28, 95% CI: 0.18–0.40).[60]

Overall, a positive SLR was present in 70% to 98% of patients with a lumbar disc pathology confirmed operatively.[80,81,83–91] The sensitivity of the test ranges from 72% to 97% whereas specificity is between 11% and 66%.[81,83,86,92–94] A systemic review and meta-analysis by Deville and colleagues[95] compiled data from numerous studies[80,81,83,86–88,93,94,96–102] evaluating the SLR test with surgery as reference standard. The results of the pooled data of these studies revealed the pooled sensitivity for the SLR test was 91% (95% CI 0.82–0.94), and the pooled specificity 26%[95] (95% CI 0.16–0.38). Although frequently regarded as the same test, Supik and Broom[103] differentiated the two (SLR as pain with any leg raise compared with positive Lasegue with 10–15° with addition of ankle dorsiflexion). In their study, the SLR was positive in 96% compared with 71% with the Lasegue maneuver.[103] Regarding the SLR's ability to predict the presence of pathology, it was found to have a positive predictive value of 67% and a negative predictive value of 57%.[104]

There have been evaluations regarding variations of the SLR, seated versus supine. The sensitivity of the supine SLR test was 67% compared with a sensitivity of 41% of the seated SLR test, concluding that the traditional supine SLR test is more sensitive in reproducing leg pain than the seated SLR test in patients presenting with signs of and symptoms consistent with lumbar radiculopathy as well as MRI evidence of nerve root compression.[105] Also, there is a recent study with results demonstrating that the SLR has a higher specificity than sensitivity in comparing it with the slump test. The slump test was found to be more sensitive, 84%, than the SLR, 52%, in the patients with lumbar disc herniations. However, the SLR was found to be a slightly more specific test (89%) than the slump test (83%).[82]

A positive SLR test can also help in determining the location of the disc herniations, as noted by Spangfort[83] while studying 2504 lumbar disc herniation surgeries.

A positive SLR was noted in 96% to 98% of the patients with herniations from L4 to S1 as compared with only 73% of patients with disc pathology from L1 to L4.

Recent literature also evaluated the validity of SLR in self-reported disability (Roland-Morris Disability Questionnaire [RMDQ]) after stratification by sex, and revealed that compared with the finger to floor test, the SLR was of less value as an indicator of self-reported disability after stratification, especially for men.[106] Nadler and colleagues[107] also evaluated whether documentation of a positive SLR was influenced by insurance coverage. In this retrospective study, the investigators evaluated the presence of positive unilateral or bilateral SLR in patients with personal injury or worker's compensation. The study revealed that a positive finding was 7.4 to 105.1 times more likely in the personal injury group, and concluded that several factors including an added incentive to treat, poor knowledge of proper interpretation of the SLR test, and/or an increased exaggeration of symptoms may have contributed to these findings.[107]

Overall, the diagnostic accuracy of the SLR test is valuable in the evaluation of lumbar radicular pain; however, it may be limited by its low specificity.

Crossed straight leg raise

The crossed straight leg raise (CSLR) was initially described in 1901 by Fajersztajn[108] after completing a cadaveric study. During this study it was noted the while performing the SLR the movement of the ipsilateral limb stretched the contralateral root by pulling laterally on the dural sac, in addition to the stretch applied to the ipsilateral root.

There have been numerous studies to assess the validity and reliability of the CSLR. The CSLR is strongly predictive of disc herniation.[109] CSLR was compared with SLR to predict the presence of disc herniation on physical examination. In this study, CSLR was positive in 97% of patients as compared with 64% with SLR alone.[110] Similarly, Andersson and Deyo[104] demonstrated that CSLR had a high positive predictive value of 79% and negative predictive value of 44%.[104] When evaluating the presence of herniations at surgery, the study by Kosteljanetz and colleagues[81] revealed that 19 of 20 positive patients had correlative findings. Overall, the prevalence of the CSLR ranged from 83% to 86%,[81,83,94,110] whereas the prevalence of CSLR in patients with lumbar disc herniations ranged between 23% and 60%.[88,89,91]

Regarding sensitivity and specificity, the crossed Lasegue was found to be 100% specific with a low sensitivity.[84,85] Andersson and Deyo[104] demonstrated that the CSLR had a higher specificity (85%–100%) and a lower sensitivity (23%–42%) as compared with the SLR when reviewing various studies.[81,83,94,104,110] The same findings were collected in pooled data by Deville and colleagues[95] and also revealed a low sensitivity (29%) and high specificity (88%). A recent Cochrane review by van der Windt and colleagues[60] provided a similar conclusion, with CSLR showing high specificity (pooled estimate 0.90, 95% CI: 0.85–0.94) with consistently low sensitivity (pooled estimate 0.28, 95% CI: 0.22–0.35).[60]

In addition, the CSLR can be useful in predicting treatment outcomes in surgical and conservative management between patients. A positive CSLR has been proven to predict poor prognosis of conservative management[111] as well as those who would have positive outcomes with surgical intervention.[96,109]

Bowstring sign

The bowstring sign, or the posterior tibial nerve sign, was originally described by Gower in 1888.[112] On elicitation of a positive SLR, further provocative testing is performed by flexion of the leg and the application of pressure in the popliteal fossa.

Reproduction of symptoms by compression of the popliteal fossa was noted to be anatomically correlated with the stretch of the sciatic nerve.[112]

There is limited literature on the sensitivity of the bowstring sign. In a study of 50 perioperative patients with clinical and radiographic evidence of disc herniation,[103] initial physical examination included evaluation of sciatic tension signs using the SLR, CSLR, Lasegue sign, and the bowstring sign. The presence of lumbar disc herniation was confirmed radiographically. Intraoperatively, the 50 patients were assessed for anatomic location of disc herniation and the presence of disc protrusion or extrusion. The bowstring sign was positive in 71% of the patients with disc pathology confirmed intraoperatively.[103] At this point, there is insufficient evidence regarding the clinical usefulness of the bowstring sign for the evaluation of lumbar radiculopathy.

Slump test

The slump test was originally described as the reproduction of sciatic pain in a seated individual, with knee extension combined with flexion of the trunk and cervical spine, by Cyriax[113] in 1942. A more recent description of the test modifies the test into a series of 3 stages.[114] In Stage 1, the patient will initiate trunk flexion with the arms behind the back while the examiner applies pressure to the back. Neck flexion will be added in Stage 2 with examiner pressure added to neck flexion. In Stage 3, the patient will maintain neck and trunk flexion, but will also extend the knee, followed by dorsiflexion of the ankle.[114] This test differs from the seated SLR,[105,115] which focuses on only the third stage of the slump test.

In a prospective case-control study of 75 patients with complaints suggestive of lumbar disc herniation,[82] 38 patients had signs of herniation demonstrated by MRI, whereas control patients (n = 37) did not have disc bulges or herniations on MRI. Both the slump and SLR tests were performed in all 75 patients. The slump test was found to be more sensitive (84%) than the SLR test (52%) in the patients with lumbar disc herniations. However, the SLR was found to be a slightly more specific test (89%) than the slump test (83%). The slump test might be used more frequently as a sensitive physical examination tool in patients with symptoms of lumbar disc herniations.[82]

Overall, there is limited scientific evidence evaluating the validity of the slump test; however, there is no current literature on its reliability. The recent literature suggests that there is a high specificity and sensitivity, but more studies should be conducted to further evaluate the slump test.

Ankle dorsiflexion test (Braggard sign)

The Braggard sign or ankle dorsiflexion test has been described in several different ways. Historically, it was first described by Fajersztajn[108] when adding ankle dorsiflexion and neck flexion to further provoke radicular pain by increasing the tension on the nerve root. A positive finding with this test typically causes pain indicative of lumbosacral/sciatic nerve involvement. A positive sign is elicited when pain radiates down the back of the buttock, thigh and, in extreme cases, calf and bottom of the foot after dorsiflexion of the ankle. This test indicates a disc lesion or subluxation ranging from the fourth lumbar vertebra down to the third sacral segment. Macrae and Wright[78] describe the standard variation that involves elevating the leg to the point of pain provocation, then lowering the limb until the pain resolves followed by ankle dorsiflexion. If the dorsiflexion causes pain, this is felt to be a positive finding.[78]

There is limited literature regarding assessing the effectiveness of the Braggard sign. A study by Stankovic and colleagues[116] compared the slump test in patients with and without disc pathology. A positive sign was found in 94.2% of patients with frank disc herniation, 78% of disc bulges, and 75% without any disc pathology. At present, more research should be conducted to fully evaluate the role of the Braggard sign in the assessment of lumbar radiculopathy.

Kemp sign

The Kemp sign is described as pain that radiates down the sciatic nerve on the side toward which the patient is bending, with a positive finding suggesting disc involvement.[117] There are no studies in the literature evaluating the validity or reliability of this sign.

Flip sign

The flip test is commonly performed in patients with sciatica to confirm nerve root tension, or otherwise, evidenced by a restricted supine SLR. Passive extension of the knee with the patient in the erect position and the hip flexed is reported to cause a sudden falling or flipping back of the trunk.[118]

There is limited literature evaluating the validity and reliability of the flip sign in its ability to assess lumbar radicular symptoms. Sixty-seven patients with sciatica and MRI scans confirming disc protrusion and nerve root compression underwent the flip test.[118] A third of the patients did not have any pain, 39% felt pain on full extension of the knee, and 28% resisted full extension of the knee due to pain. Only one-third of patients demonstrated a "flip." All patients with a supine SLR below 45° showed a painful response, so the flip test is a useful check of nerve root tension but only for patients with supine SLRs below 45°. The most reliable response was not a "flip" but the demonstration of pain on extension of the knee, constituting a seated SLR.[118]

Negative extension sign

The negative extension sign[119] is described as the patient's ability to achieve full passive lumbar extension. This sign may be useful as a clinical predictor in the evaluation of lumbar radiculopathy in patients with herniated nucleus pulposus (HNP) and potential response to conservative management.

Alexander and colleagues[119] evaluated the efficacy of conservative management based on a negative extension sign. The study revealed a favorable response to nonoperative therapy for radicular symptoms in patients with an HNP in 91% of the cases at long-term follow-up. At present, there is insufficient literature regarding the negative extension sign to make a significant contribution to the assessment of a patient with suspected radiculopathy.

Femoral nerve stretch test

The femoral nerve stretch test (FNST) is most commonly described as being performed with a prone patient undergoing passive flexion of the knee by the examiner. A positive finding is determined by the elicitation of pain in the back and the anterior aspect of the thigh correlating to the patient's typical pain distribution. This test was first described by Wassermann[120] in 1918 while evaluating soldiers who complained of anterior thigh and shin pain, and the absence of provocation with the Lasegue sign.[120] There is some variance in the presumed pathophysiology; however, it is thought that the test provides a stretch of the L2-L4 nerve roots and that the traction forces cause movement of these nerve roots.[121,122]

Due to the low frequency of upper lumbar disc herniations, the presence of the symptoms is less commonly seen. With studies demonstrating positive findings in 84% to 95% of patients with upper lumbar disc pathology, it is felt that the FNST in likely the single best screening test for upper lumbar radiculopathy.[123,124,125] There may be increased sensitivity with this test with the addition of hip extension[114] or extension of the spine.[126]

A recent study by Suri and colleagues[59] evaluated both FNST and crossed FNST with other physical examination findings. The FNST was predictive in determining midlumbar impingement either alone or when combined with either patellar reflex testing or the sit-to-stand test. Regarding prediction of a level-specific impingement, a positive FNST best correlated pathology at L3.[59] Additional studies evaluating a level-specific impingement or disc pathology level provided strong correlation, with a positive FNST at L3/4[121] and L4/5.[123]

There are no studies evaluating predicting treatment outcomes with a positive FNST and either conservative or surgical management.

Crossed femoral nerve test

In comparison with FNST data, there is limited literature regarding the crossed femoral nerve test (CFNT). Historically, it was first described by Cyriax[113] in 1947, and is felt to produce the same radicular symptoms as the FNST when providing the same provocative maneuver on the contralateral limb. The proposed pathology is that the extension of the limb will put traction on the upper lumbar nerve roots by stretching the psoas and quadriceps femoris.[122]

Until recently, the only literature evaluating the CFNT was a report on 2 cases of upper lumbar radiculopathy and the presence of a positive finding with CFNT.[127,128] However, the recent study by Suri and colleagues[59] evaluated the CFNT for mid and low lumbar nerve root impingement. The study revealed that the CFNT was predictive of midlumbar impingement and L4 level-specific impingement alone and when combined with other tests; however, it did not correlate with low-level impingement.[59]

At present, more evidence is necessary regarding the validity and reliability of the CFNT in the clinical evaluation of lumbar radiculopathy.

Nonorganic signs

There are nonorganic signs on physical examination that can be used as a simple clinical screen to help identify patients who require more detailed psychological assessment. Waddell and colleagues[115] first described these findings in a study of 350 patients with low back pain. These nonorganic signs are distinguishable from the standard clinical signs of physical pathology and correlate with other psychological data. By helping to separate the physical from the nonorganic, they clarify the assessment of purely physical pathologic conditions.

Waddell and colleagues[115] described 5 distinct findings: tenderness, simulation, distraction, regional, and overreaction.

- Regional: Widespread distribution of symptoms divergent from accepted neuroanatomy or physiology
- Overreaction: Disproportionate verbalization, facial expressions, muscle tension, tremors, collapsing, or sweating
- Simulation: During formal examination the test produces symptoms, then the test is simulated without being performed, and elicits pain suggesting a nonorganic sign
- Tenderness: Superficial—discomfort with light touch over a diffuse area. Nonanatomic—deep tenderness over a widespread area
- Distraction: Positive finding demonstrated in the traditional manner, then assessed again in another manner or when the patient is distracted.

Three or more positive findings during physical examination are suggestive of physical findings without anatomic cause. There is a correlation with potential psychological overlay; however, this is not suggestive of malingering. Overall, it is a reliable test that is 80% reproducible with a kappa coefficient between 0.55 and 0.71. The nonorganic signs are a helpful screen for the clinician to identify patients who may benefit from a more detailed psychological evaluation.[89,104,115,127–129]

Hoover

First described by Arieff in 1961,[130,131] the Hoover sign may be useful in assessing the patient's voluntary effort during the physical examination. With the patient supine, the physician will hold the patient's heels and instruct the patient to perform an active SLR. It is described that if the patient is providing a voluntary effort to raise the leg, then an increased downward pressure should be felt in the contralateral heel. There are no studies in the literature evaluating the validity or reliability of this sign.

SUMMARY

Physical examination of the patient with suspected radiculopathy needs to be thorough and complete to make the most accurate diagnosis. Knowledge of the literature related to the specific physical examination findings is imperative for the clinician to make the most accurate assessment and to guide the further diagnosis and treatment.

Based on the evidence-based literature, there are several physical examination findings that are extremely helpful in the evaluation of cervical and lumbar radiculopathy. In the examination of cervical radiculopathy, besides the Spurling test, there is limited research on the validity and reliability as regards the provocative tests. Of the other tests, the shoulder abduction relief sign, ULTT, and neck distractions sign have evidence that suggest utility in the evaluation process. Comparatively, there is significantly more evidence-based literature on the lumbar spine. There is a prolific amount of evidence regarding SLR and CSLR. Both have clinical significance in the evaluation of lumbar radiculopathy, with SLR having a high sensitivity and low sensitivity, and the CSLR having a high specificity and low sensitivity. Until recently there has been very limited evidence-based research on other lumbar provocative tests; however, with these new contributions there is a better understanding of the utility of these tests.

Overall, the physical examination is the cornerstone of the evaluation and treatment of radiculopathy, and thorough knowledge of the evidence-based literature will become extremely beneficial in maximizing patient care, particularly in the light of health care reform.

REFERENCES

1. Greenberg SA. The history of dermatome mapping. Arch Neurol 2003;60: 126–31.
2. Marzo JM, Simmons EH, Kallen F. Intradural connections between adjacent cervical spinal roots. Spine 1987;12(10):964–8.
3. Foerster O. The dermatomes in man. Brain 1933;56:1–39.
4. Brazier MA, Watkins AL, Michelsen JJ. Electromyography in differential diagnosis of ruptured cervical disk. Arch Neurol Psychiatry 1946;56:651–8.
5. Brendler SJ. The human cervical myotomes: functional anatomy studied at operation. J Neurosurg 1968;28:105–11.
6. Levin KH, Maggiano HJ, Wilbourn AJ. Cervical radiculopathies: comparison of surgical and EMG localization of single-root lesions. Neurology 1996;46:1022–5.

7. Tsao BE, Levin KH, Bodner RA. Comparison of surgical and electrodiagnostic findings in single root lumbosacral radiculopathies. Muscle Nerve 2003;27: 60–4.
8. Phillips LH, Park TS. Electrophysiologic mapping of the segmental anatomy of the muscle of the lower extremity. Muscle Nerve 1991;14:1213–8.
9. Lauder TD, Dillingham TR, Andary M, et al. Effect of history and exam in predicting electrodiagnostic outcome among patients with suspected lumbosacral radiculopathy. Am J Phys Med Rehabil 2000;79:60–8.
10. Levin KH. Electrodiagnostic approach to the patient with suspected radiculopathy. Neurol Clin 2002;20:397–421.
11. Eubanks JD. Cervical radiculopathy: nonoperative management of neck pain and radicular symptoms. Am Fam Physician 2010;81(1):33–40.
12. Kuijper B, Tans JT, Schimsheimer RJ, et al. Degenerative cervical radiculopathy: diagnosis and conservative treatment. A review. Eur J Neurol 2009;16(1):15–20.
13. Rubenstein SM, van Tulder M. A best-evidence review of diagnostic procedures for neck and low-back pain. Best Pract Res Clin Rheumatol 2008;22(3):471–82.
14. Rubenstein SM, Pool JJ, van Tulder MW, et al. A systematic review of the diagnostic accuracy of provocative tests of the neck for diagnosing cervical radiculopathy. Eur Spine J 2007;16(3):307–19.
15. Nordin M, Carragee EJ, Hogg-Johnson S, et al. Assessment of neck pain and its associated disorders: results of the Bone and Joint Decade 2000–2010 Task Force on Neck Pain and its Associated Disorders. Spine (Phila Pa 1976) 2008;33(Suppl 4):S101–22.
16. Guzman J, Haldeman S, Carroll LJ, et al. Clinical practice implications of the Bone and Joint Decade 2000-2010 Task Force on Neck Pain and its Associated Disorders: from concepts and findings to recommendations. Spine (Phila Pa 1976) 2008;33(Suppl 4):S199–213.
17. Abbed KM, Coumans JV. Cervical radiculopathy: pathophysiology, presentation, and clinical evaluation. Neurosurgery 2007;60(1 Supp1 1):S28–34.
18. Malanga GA, Landes P, Nadler SF. Provocative tests in cervical spine examination: historical basis and scientific analyses. Pain Physician 2003;6(2):199–205.
19. Landes P, Malanga GA, Nadler SF, et al. Musculoskeletal physical examination: an evidence-based approach. In: Malanga GA, Nadler SF, editors. Physical examination of the cervical spine. Elsevier Mosby; 2006. p. 33–57, chapter 3.
20. Douglass AB, Bope ET. Evaluation and treatment of posterior neck pain in family practice. J Am Board Fam Pract 2004;17(Suppl):S13–22.
21. Wainner RS, Fritz JM, Irrgang JJ, et al. Reliability and diagnostic accuracy of the clinical examination and patient self-report measures for cervical radiculopathy. Spine (Phila Pa 1976) 2003;28(1):52–62.
22. Manifold SG, McCann PD. Cervical radiculitis and shoulder disorders. Clin Orthop Relat Res 1999;368:105–13.
23. Malanga GA. The diagnosis and treatment of cervical radiculopathy. Med Sci Sports Exerc 1997;29(Suppl 7):S236–45.
24. Ellenberg MR, Honet JC, Treanor WJ. Cervical radiculopathy. Arch Phys Med Rehabil 1994;75(3):342–52.
25. Ellenberg MR, Honet JC. Clinical pearls in cervical radiculopathy. Phys Med Rehabil Clin N Am 1996;7:487–508.
26. Hong CZ, Lee S, Lum P. Cervical radiculopathy. Clinical, radiographic and EMG findings. Orthop Rev 1986;15(7):433–9.
27. Fager CA. Identification and management of radiculopathy. Neurosurg Clin N Am 1993;4(1):1–12.

28. Spurling RG, Scoville WB. Lateral rupture of the cervical intervertebral discs: a common cause of shoulder and arm pain. Surg Gynecol Obstet 1944;78: 350–8.
29. Shah KC, Rajshekhar V. Reliability of diagnosis of soft cervical disc prolapse using Spurling's test. Br J Neurosurg 2004;18(5):480–3.
30. Viikari-Juntura E. Interexaminer reliability of observations in physical examination of the neck. Phys Ther 1987;67:1526–32.
31. Viikari-Juntura E, Porras M, Laasonen EM. Validity of clinical tests in the diagnosis of root compression in cervical disease. Spine (Phila Pa 1976) 1989;14: 253–7.
32. Tong HC, Haig AJ, Yamaka K. The Spurling test and cervical radiculopathy. Spine (Phila Pa 1976) 2002;27(2):156–9.
33. Sandmark H, Nisell R. Validity of five common manual neck pain provoking tests. Scand J Rehabil Med 1995;27(3):131–6.
34. Uchihara T, Furukawa T, Tsukagoshi H. Compression of brachial plexus as a diagnosis test of cervical cord lesion. Spine (Phila Pa 1976) 1994;19: 2170–3.
35. Lhermitte JJ. Les forms douloureuses de commotion de la moelle epiniere. Rev Neurol 1920;36:257–62.
36. Lhermitte JJ, Pollak NM. Les douleurs à type discharge éléctrique consécutives à la flexion cephalique dans la sclérose en plaques. Un cas de la sclérose multiple. Rev Neurol (Paris) 1924;2:56–7.
37. Lhermitte JJ. Multiple sclerosis. Arch Neurol Psychiatry 1929;22:5–8.
38. Marie P, Chatelin C. Sur certains symtomes vraisemblablement d'orogine radiculaire chez les blessed du crane. Rev Neurol 1917;31:336.
39. Babinski J, Dubois R. Douleurs a forme de decharge electrique, consecutives aux traumatismes de la nuque. Presse Med 1918;26:64.
40. Davidson RI, Dunn EJ, Metzmaker JN. The shoulder abduction test in the diagnosis of radicular pain in cervical extradural compressive monoradiculopathies. Spine (Phila Pa 1976) 1981;6(5):441–6.
41. Magee DJ. Cervical spine. In: Magee DJ, editor. Orthopedic physical assessment. 3rd editon. Philadelphia: WB Saunders; 1997.
42. BeattyRM, Fowler FD, Hanson EJ. The abducted arm as a sign of ruptured cervical disc. Neurosugery 1987;21(5):731–2.
43. Fast A, Parikh S, Marin EL. The shoulder abduction relief sign in cervical radiculopathy. Arch Phys Med Rehabil 1989;70:402–3.
44. Quintner JL. A study of upper limb pain and paraesthesiae following neck injury in motor vehicle accidents: assessment of the brachial plexus tension test of Elvey. Br J Rheumatol 1989;28(6):528–33.
45. Elvey RL. The investigation of arm pain: signs of adverse responses to the physical examination of the brachial plexus, related tissues. In: Boyling JD, Palastanga N, editors. Grieve's modern manual therapy. 2nd edition. New York (NY): Churchill Livingstone; 1995. p. 577–85.
46. Bendheim OL. On the history of Hoffmann's sign. Bull Inst Hist Med 1937;5: 684–5.
47. Cooper MJ. Mechanical factors governing the Tromner reflex. Arch Neurol Psychiatry 1933;30:166–9.
48. Curschmann H. Uber die diagnostiche bedeutung des Babinskischen phanomens im prauramischen zustand. Munch Med Wochenschr 1911;58:2054–7.
49. Echols DH. The Hoffmann sign: its incidence in university students. J Nerv Ment Dis 1936;84:427–31.

50. Keyser TS. Hoffmann's sign or the "digital reflex". J Nerv Ment Dis 1916;44: 51–62.
51. Madonick MJ. Statistical control studies in neurology. III: The Hoffmann sign. Arch Neurol Psychiatry 1952;68:109–15.
52. Pitfield RL. The Hoffmann reflex: a simple way of reinforcing it and other reflexes. J Nerv Ment Dis 1929;69:252–8.
53. Schneck JM. The unilateral Hoffman reflex. J Nerv Ment Dis 1946;104:597–8.
54. Tromner E. Euber sehnen-respective muskelreflexe und die merkmale ihrer schwachung und steigerung. Berl Klin Wchnschr 1913;50:1712–5.
55. Sung RD, Wang JC. Correlation between a positive Hoffman's reflex and cervical pathology in asymptomatic individuals. Spine (Phila Pa 1976) 2001;26:67–70.
56. Denno JJ, Meadows GR. Early diagnosis of cervical spondylotic myelopathy: a useful clinical sign. Spine (Phila Pa 1976) 1991;16:1353–5.
57. Glaser JA, et al. Cervical cord compression and the Hoffman's sign. Presented at the 14th Annual Meeting of the North American Spine Society. Chicago (IL), October 21, 1999.
58. Raaf J. Surgery for cervical rib and scalenus anticus syndrome. JAMA 1965; 157:219.
59. Suri P, Rainville J, Katz JN, et al. The accuracy of the physical examination for the diagnosis of midlumbar and low lumbar nerve root impingement. Spine (Phila Pa 1976) 2011;36(1):63–73.
60. van der Windt DA, Simons E, Riphagen II, et al. Physical examination for lumbar radiculopathy due to disc herniation in patients with low-back pain. Cochrane Database Syst Rev 2010;2:CD007431.
61. Coster S, de Bruijn SF, Tavy DL. Diagnostic value of history, physical examination and needle electromyography in diagnosing lumbosacral radiculopathy. J Neurol 2010;257(3):332–7.
62. Last AR, Hulbert K. Chronic low back pain: evaluation and management. Am Fam Physician 2009;79(12):1067–74.
63. Chou R, Qaseem A, Snow V, et al. Diagnosis and treatment of low back pain: a joint clinical practice guideline from the American College of Physicians and the American Pain Society. Ann Intern Med 2007;147(7):478–91.
64. Miller KJ. Physical assessment of lower extremity radiculopathy and sciatica. J Chiropr Med 2007;6(2):75–82.
65. van Rijn JC, Klemetso N, Reitsma JB, et al. Symptomatic and asymptomatic abnormalities in patients with lumbosacral radicular syndrome: clinical examination compared with MRI. Clin Neurol Neurosurg 2006;108(6):553–7.
66. Vroomen PC, de Krom MC, Wilmink JT, et al. Diagnostic value of history and physical examination in patients suspected of lumbosacral nerve root compression. J Neurol Neurosurg Psychiatry 2002;72(5):630–4.
67. Patel AT, Ogle AA. Diagnosis and management of acute low back pain. Am Fam Physician 2000;61(6):1779–86, 1789–90.
68. Humphreys SC, Eck JC. Clinical evaluation and treatment options for herniated lumbar disc. Am Fam Physician 1999;59(3):575–82, 587–8.
69. Dvorak J. Epidemiology, physical examination, and neurodiagnostics. Spine (Phila Pa 1976) 1998;23(24):2663–73.
70. Lazarevič LK. Ischias postica cotunnii: a contribution to the differential diagnosis. Srp Arh Celok Lek 1880;7:23–35 [Serbian Archives of Medicine].
71. Lazarevič LK. Ischias postica Cotunnii. Ein Beitrag zu deren Differential-Diagnose. Allgemeine Wiener medizinische Zeitung 1884;29:425–6.
72. Frost JJ. Contribution à l'ètude clinique de la sciatique. Thèse No 1881;33.

73. Karbowski K, Radanov BP. Historical perspective: the history of the discovery of the sciatica stretching phenomenon. Spine (Phila Pa 1976) 1995;20:1315–7.
74. Inman VT, Saunders JB. The clinico-anatomical aspects of the lumbosacral region. Radiology 1942;38:669–78.
75. Falconer MA, McGeorge M, Begg AC. Observations on the cause and mechanism of symptom production in sciatica and low back pain. J Neurol Neurosurg Psychiatry 1948;11:13–26.
76. Goddard MD, Reid JD. Movements induced by straight leg raising in the lumbosacral roots, nerves, and plexus and in the intrapelvic section of the sciatic nerve. J Neurol Neurosurg Psychiatry 1965;28:12–8.
77. Loebl WY. Measurement of spinal posture and range of spinal movement. Ann Phys Med 1967;9:103–1107.
78. Macrae IF, Wright V. Measurements of back movement. Ann Rheum Dis 1969; 28:584–9.
79. Fahrni WH. Observation on straight leg raising with special reference to nerve root adhesions. Can J Surg 1966;9:44–8.
80. Shiqing X, Quanzhi Z, Dehao F. Significance of the straight leg raising test in the diagnosis and clinical evaluation of lower lumbar intervertebral disc protrusion. J Bone Joint Surg Am 1987;69:517–22.
81. Kosteljanetz M, Bang F, Schmidt-Olsen S. The clinical significance of straight leg raising (Lasegue's sign) in the diagnosis of prolapsed lumbar disc: interobserver variation and correlation with surgical findings. Spine (Phila Pa 1976) 1988;13:393–5.
82. Majlesi J, Togay H, Unalan H, et al. The sensitivity and specificity of the Slump and the Straight Leg Raising tests in patients with lumbar disc herniation. J Clin Rheumatol 2008;14(2):87–91.
83. Spangfort E. Lasegue's sign in patients with lumbar disc herniation. Acta Orthop Scand 1971;42:459–60.
84. Thomas M, Grant N, Marshall J. Surgical treatment of low backache and sciatica. Lancet 1983;2:1437–9.
85. Thomas E, Silman AJ, Papageorgiou AC, et al. Association between measures of spinal mobility and low back pain: an analysis of new attenders in primary care. Spine (Phila Pa 1976) 1998;23:343–7.
86. Kosteljanetz M, Esperen JO, Halburt H, et al. Predictive value of clinical and surgical findings in patients with lumbago-sciatica; a prospective study (part 1). Acta Neurochir (Wien) 1984;73:67–76.
87. Jonsson B, Stromqvist B. The straight leg raising test and the severity of symptoms in lumbar disc herniation. Spine (Phila Pa 1976) 1995;20:27–30.
88. Jonsson B, Stromqvist B. Symptoms and signs in degeneration of the lumbar spine: a prospective, consecutive study of 300 operated patients. J Bone Joint Surg Br 1993;75:381–5.
89. Vucetic N, Svensson O. Physical signs in lumbar disc hernia. Clin Orthop 1996; 333:192–201.
90. Kortelainen P, Puranen J, Koivisto E, et al. Symptoms and signs of sciatica and their relation to the localization of the lumbar disc herniation. Spine (Phila Pa 1976) 1985;10:88–92.
91. Spengler DM, Ouellette AE, Battie M, et al. Elective discectomy for herniation of lumbar disc. J Bone Joint Surg Am 1990;72:230–7.
92. Charnely J. Orthopaedic signs in the diagnosis of disc protrusion, with special reference to the straight leg raising test. Lancet 1951;260:186–92.
93. Hakelius A. Prognosis in sciatica. Acta Orthop Scand 1970;129(Suppl):1–70.

94. Hakelius A, Hindmarsh J. The comparative reliability of preoperative diagnostic methods in lumbar disc surgery. Acta Orthop Scand 1972;43:234–8.
95. Deville WL, van der Windt DA, Dzaferagic A, et al. The test of Lasegue: a systematic review of the accuracy in diagnosing herniated discs. Spine (Phila Pa 1976) 2000;25:1140–7.
96. Edgar MA, Park WM. Induced pain patterns of passive straight leg raising in lower lumbar disc protrusion. J Bone Joint Surg Br 1974;56:658–66.
97. Kerr RS, Cadoux-Hudson TA, Adams CB. The value of accurate clinical assessment in the surgical management of the lumbar disc protrusion. J Neurol Neurosurg Psychiatry 1988;51:169–73.
98. Knuttson B. Comparative value of electromyographic, myelographic, and clinical-neurological examinations in the diagnosis of lumbar root compression syndrome. Acta Orthop Scand 1961;49(Suppl):1–34.
99. Gudjian ES, Webster JE, Ostrowski AZ, et al. Herniated lumbar intervertebral discs: an analysis of 1176 operated cases. J Trauma 1961;1:158–76.
100. Aronson HA, Dunsmore RH. Herniated upper lumbar discs. J Bone Joint Surg Am 1963;45:311–7.
101. Albeck MJ. A critical assessment of clinical diagnosis of disc herniation in patients with monoradicular sciatica. Acta Neurochir (Wien) 1996;138:40–4.
102. Hirsch C, Nachemson A. The reliability of lumbar disk surgery. Clin Orthop 1963; 29:189–95.
103. Supik LF, Broom MJ. Sciatic tension signs and lumbar disc herniation. Spine (Phila Pa 1976) 1994;19:1066–9.
104. Andersson GB, Deyo RA. History and physical examination in patients with herniated lumbar discs. Spine (Phila Pa 1976) 1996;21(Suppl 24):10–85.
105. Rabin A, Gerszten PC, Karausky P, et al. The sensitivity of the seated straight-leg raise test compared with the supine straight-leg raise test in patients presenting with magnetic resonance imaging evidence of lumbar nerve root compression. Arch Phys Med Rehabil 2007;88(7):840–3.
106. Ekedahl KH, Jonsson B, Frobell RB. Validity of the fingertip-to-floor test and straight leg raising test in patients with acute and subacute low back pain: a comparison by sex and radicular pain. Arch Phys Med Rehabil 2010;91(8): 1243–7.
107. Nadler SF, Malanga GA, Ciccone DS. Positive straight-leg raising in lumbar radiculopathy: is documentation affected by insurance coverage? Arch Phys Med Rehabil 2004;85(8):1336–8.
108. Fajersztajn J. Ueber das gekreuzte ischiaphanomen. Wien Klin Wochenschr 1901;14:41–7.
109. Woodhall B, Hayes G. The well leg raising test of Fajerstajn in the diagnosis of ruptured lumbar inter-vertebral disc. J Bone Joint Surg Am 1950;32: 786–92.
110. Hudgins WR. The crossed straight leg raising test: a diagnostic sign of herniated disc. J Occup Med 1979;21:407–8.
111. Khuffash B, Porter RW. Cross leg pain and trunk list. Spine (Phila Pa 1976) 1989; 14:602–3.
112. Cram RH. A sign of the sciatic nerve root pressure. J Bone Joint Surg Br 1953; 25:192–5.
113. Cyriax J. Perineuritis. Br Med J 1942;1:578–80.
114. Geraci MC, Alleva JT. Physical examination of the spine and its functional kinetic chain. In: Cole AJ, Herring SA, editors. The low back pain handbook. Philadelphia: Hanley & Belfus; 1996. p. 60.

115. Waddell G, McCulloch JA, Kummel E, et al. Nonorganic physical signs in low-back pain. Spine (Phila Pa 1976) 1980;5:117–25.
116. Stankovic R, Johnell O, Maly P, et al. Use of lumbar extension, slump test, physical and neurological examination in the evaluation of patients with suspected herniated nucleus pulposus: a prospective clinical study. Man Ther 1999;4(1):25–32.
117. Walsh MJ. Evaluation of orthopedic testing of the low back for nonspecific lower back pain. J Manipulative Physiol Ther 1998;21(4):232–6.
118. Summers B, Mishra V, Jones JM. The flip test: a reappraisal. Spine (Phila Pa 1976) 2009;34(15):1585–9.
119. Alexander AH, Jones AM, Rosenbaum DH Jr. Nonoperative management of herniated nucleus pulposus: patient selection by the extension sign. Long-term follow-up. Orthop Rev 1992;21(2):181–8.
120. Wassermann S. Euber ein neues Schenkelnersyptom nebstr Bemerkungen zur Diagnostik der Schenkelnerverkrankungen. Ditsch Z Nervenbeilk 1918/19;43: 140–3.
121. Estridge MN, Rothe SA, Johnson NG. The femoral stretching test: a valuable sign in diagnosing upper lumbar disc herniation. J Neurosurg 1982;57:813–7.
122. Dyck P. The femoral nerve traction test with lumbar disc protrusions. Surg Neurol 1976;6:163–6.
123. Christodoulides AN. Ipsilateral sciatica on the femoral nerve stretch test is pathognomonic of an L4/5 disc protrusion. J Bone Joint Surg Br 1989;71:88–9.
124. Abdullah AF, Wolber PG, Warfield JR, et al. Surgical management of extreme lateral lumbar disc herniations. Neurosurgery 1988;22:648–53.
125. Porchet F, Frankhauser H, de Tribolet N. Extreme lateral lumbar disc herniation: a clinical presentation of 178 patients. Acta Neurochir (Wien) 1994;127:203–9.
126. Penning L, Wolmink JT. Biomechanics of Lumbosacral dural sac: a study of flexion-extension myelography. Spine (Phila Pa 1976) 1981;6:398–408.
127. Nadler SF, Malanga GA, Stitik TP, et al. The crossed femoral nerve stretch test to improve diagnostic sensitivity for the high lumbar radiculopathy: two case reports. Arch Phys Med Rehabil 2001;82:522–3.
128. Waddell G, Main CJ, Morris EW, et al. Normality and reliability in the clinical assessment of backache. Br Med J (Clin Res Ed) 1982;284:1519–23.
129. Waddell G, Somerville D, Henderson I, et al. Objective clinical evaluation of physical impairment in chronic low back pain. Spine (Phila Pa 1976) 1992;17: 617–28.
130. Arieff AJ. The Hoover sign: an objective sign of pain and/or weakness in the back or lower extremities. Trans Am Neurol Assoc 1961;86:191.
131. Arieff AJ, Tigay EL, Kurtz JF, et al. The Hoover sign. An objective-sign of pain and/or weakness in the back or lower extremities. Arch Neurol 1961;5:673–8.
132. Barz T, Melloh M, Staub LP, et al. Nerve root sedimentation sign: evaluation of a new radiological sign in lumbar spinal stenosis. Spine (Phila PA 1976) 2010; 35(8):892–7.
133. Freynhagen R, Rolke R, Baron R, et al. Pseudoradicular and radicular low-back pain—a disease continuum rather than different entities? Answers from quantitative sensory testing. Pain 2008;135(1–2):65–74.
134. Rainville J, Noto DJ, Jouve C, et al. Assesment of forearm pronation strength in C6 and C7 radiculopathies. Spine (Phila PA 1976) 2007;32(1):72–5.
135. Haig AJ, Tzeng HM, LeBreck DB. The value of electrodiagnostic consultation for patients with upper extremity nerve complaints: a prospective comparison with the history and physical examination. Arch Phy Med Rehabil 1999;80(10): 1273–81.

Imaging in Radiculopathy

Jose Mena, MD*, Andrew L. Sherman, MD

KEYWORDS

• Diagnostic imaging • Spine • Radiculopathy • Rehabilitation

All patients presenting with signs and symptoms of lumbar radiculopathy must undergo a thorough history taking and physical examination. After reviewing the dermatomal and myotomal patterns of the condition, astute clinicians often think that they are able to make the diagnosis. Often however, the diagnosis remains unclear; it is accurate anatomically, but the underlying cause of the lesion is not confirmed or the symptoms are so severe that more information on the anatomy is required. Finally, the patient may present with red flags that suggest that the cause of their condition is not benign. Therefore, often, the next step in the diagnostic process is to order imaging studies to attempt to confirm the suspected diagnosis or rule out more serious pathologic condition.

There are several imaging examinations that are used as an extension of history taking and physical examination, including plain radiographs, magnetic resonance imaging (MRI), computed tomography (CT), CT myelogram, selective nerve root block, and bone scan.

PLAIN RADIOGRAPHS

Plain radiographs of the spine usually consist of anteroposterior and lateral views. Specialized circumstances, such as the suspicion of spondylolysis, require oblique views. Inquires into alignment and instability requires dynamic flexion/extension motion views (**Figs. 1** and **2**). Spine radiographs can also investigate whether the primary source of the spinal pain is related to malignancies, infections, instability, inflammatory spondyloarthropathies, and fractures (osteoporotic or pathologic) but with a lesser sensitivity than other imaging studies.[1] Osteophyte formation from zygapophyseal joints or severe spondylolisthesis may raise concern about nerve root impingement, but this must be confirmed by more detailed imaging, such as CT scan or MRI.[2]

Although many clinicians most often recommend radiographs as the first-line imaging study to investigate spinal pain,[3] a lot has been written about the lack of

The authors have nothing to disclose.
Department of Rehabilitation Medicine, University of Miami Miller School of Medicine, PO Box 016960 (D-461), Miami, FL 33101, USA
* Corresponding author.
E-mail address: jmena@med.miami.edu

Phys Med Rehabil Clin N Am 22 (2011) 41–57
doi:10.1016/j.pmr.2010.10.004
1047-9651/11/$ – see front matter. Published by Elsevier Inc.

pmr.theclinics.com

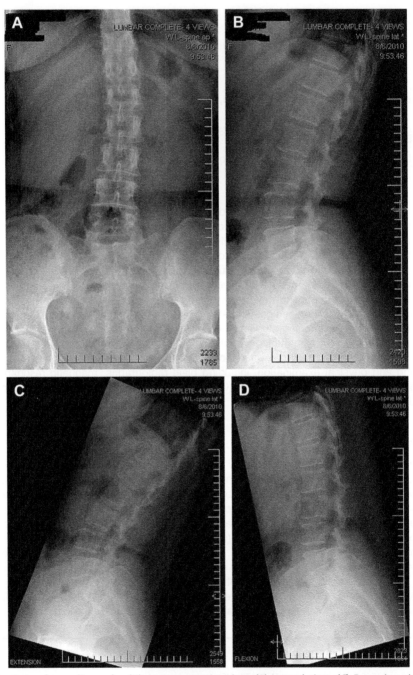

Fig. 1. Lumbar radiographs. (*A*) Anteroposterior view. (*B*) Lateral view. (*C*) Extension view. (*D*) Flexion view. Please note that there is no translation between the flexion and extension views. (*Courtesy of* the University of Miami- Miller School of Medicine.)

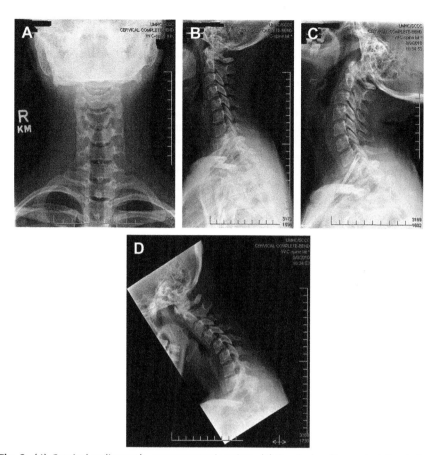

Fig. 2. (*A*) Cervical radiograph, anteroposterior view. (*B*) Cervical radiograph, lateral view. Note the anterolisthesis at C4 on C5, causing loss of the normal cervical lordosis. Dynamic flexion-extension radiographs were taken. (*C*) Cervical extension radiograph. (*D*) Cervical flexion radiograph. Note the minimal retrolisthesis at C4 on C5 estimated to be 2 to 3 mm compared with the extension radiograph of the same patient. (*Courtesy of* the University of Miami- Miller School of Medicine.)

effectiveness of radiographs to make relevant diagnoses. In 1987, the Quebec Task Force in proposed a classification to emphasize simple clinical criteria based on history taking (eg, location of symptoms, duration, and work status), physical examination findings, radiological test results, and response to treatment. This task force classified activity-related spinal disorders into 11 categories and subdivided these categories according to the working status during evaluation along with the duration of symptoms. For patients with radicular symptoms, the Quebec Task Force classification was highly associated with the severity of symptoms and the probability of subsequent surgical treatment. Nonsurgically treated patients in the Quebec Task Force classification categories reflecting nerve root compression had greater improvement than those with pain symptoms alone. Among surgical patients, the Quebec Task Force classification was not associated with outcome.[4,5]

The most obvious shortcoming of radiograph is the lack of ability to see soft tissue structures such as spinal disks, nerves, muscles, or ligaments. Radiographs also lack fine detail of bony structures such as small osteophytes, canal size, lateral recess diameter, and end plate irregularities, which are seen better by CT or MRI. Finally, radiographs lack specificity when it comes to the abnormalities found as published studies have revealed that many asymptomatic volunteers had the same abnormities as patients with symptoms of spinal pain.

Despite the drawbacks, the routine of performing screening radiographs at the time of initial presentation or injury remains. Typically, more advanced imaging such as MRI, CT, or bone scan is not performed on initial presentation unless a red flag is identified for the severity of symptoms requiring such an inquiry. However, because many patients with spinal pain and radiculopathy do not respond with conservative management even after weeks of medical and rehabilitation treatments, more detailed imaging becomes necessary. MRI or CT is recommended earlier in patients with severe or progressive neurologic deficits or with serious underlying conditions, such as vertebral infection, cauda equina syndrome, or cancer with spinal cord compression.[6]

MRI

MRI has become the most popular imaging modality for the investigation of spinal radiculopathy. Highly sensitive for disk, bone, and nerve abnormalities and lacking the radiation exposure of CT, MRI presents the most accurate information on the spine anatomy. MRI is the most sensitive imaging modality available to identify disk and soft tissue abnormalities in the spine. No imaging study can offer the visualization of the soft tissues in the spine such as disks, spinal nerves, and fat-related structures in as much detail (**Fig. 3**). Sheehan[7] indicates that the possible uses of MRI for low-back pain include predictive diagnostic assessment of severity, prognostic assessment of recovery, management planning, therapeutic planning, and occupational planning. Other studies, however, find the use of MRI to predict severity of symptoms or clinical outcomes to be unreliable because of the high sensitivity and low specificity of degenerative findings. For this reason, many national guidelines discourage the use of MRI in nonspecific low-back pain, although they do support its use to investigate for progressive neurologic symptoms to

1. Exclude serious pathologic conditions, such as tumors or infections
2. Correlate the level of abnormality to clinical symptoms of radiculopathy
3. Plan surgical management of spinal stenosis and radiculopathy.[7]

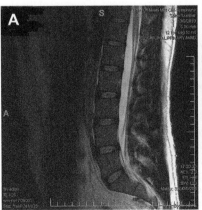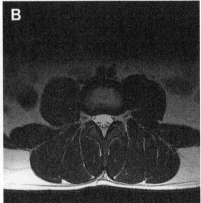

Fig. 3. (*A*) Normal sagittal T2-weighted lumbar magnetic resonance image (MRI). (*B*) Normal axial T2-weighted lumbar MRI at the level of L3-4 disk. (*Courtesy of* the University of Miami-Miller School of Medicine.)

Adding gadolinium contrast can increase the sensitivity to identify malignant causes of spinal pain, such as infection, abscess, or malignant tumor. Fat suppression imaging can increase the sensitivity for identifying stress and insufficiency fractures and hyperintense signal within the spinal cord or plexus.

Both T1- and T2-weighted pulse sequences used together comprising sagittal and axial slices of the affected area of the spine offer the greatest view of the anatomy of the spine and associated neurologic structures to include or exclude abnormality. T1-weighted images, both in the sagittal and axial planes, are useful to evaluate epidural foraminal fat, whereas T2-weighted images are useful to evaluate neural structures, disk morphology, and facet joints. When clinically indicated, gadolinium-enhanced T1 sequences obtained both in the axial and sagittal planes are useful to differentiate between disk material (herniation of the nucleus pulposus) and granulation tissue of a previous surgery or surgeries.

The high sensitivity of MRI is not only its greatest achievement and advantage but also its greatest limitation. Jensen and colleagues[8] found that on MRI examination of the lumbar spine, asymptomatic individuals without low-back pain can have disk bulges and protrusions. Jarvik and Deyo[2] noted that extrusions are rare in asymptomatic patients. Therefore, it was concluded in the study that bulges and protrusions found on MRI in people with low-back pain or even radiculopathy may be coincidental. In summary, a patient's clinical situation must be carefully evaluated in conjunction with the results of MRI (**Figs. 4–6**).[8] Other investigators have found similar findings of degenerative disks and annular tears in many asymptomatic individuals, reducing the specificity of these findings.

For the more advanced abnormalities, other investigators find a better specificity. Thornbury and colleagues[9] demonstrated a sensitivity of MRI for small herniated disks of 89% to 100% but a specificity of only 43% to 57%. In a meta-analysis, Kent and colleagues[10] demonstrated that the sensitivity of MRI for diagnosing high-grade stenosis (**Figs. 7 and 8**) was 81% to 97% and the specificity ranged from 72% to 100%. When stricter criteria for false-positive findings were used, the specificity was 93% to 100%. In addition, other investigators have found a higher specificity

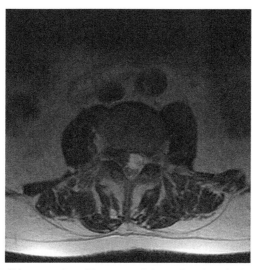

Fig. 4. A right L4-5 disk protrusion. (*Courtesy of* the University of Miami- Miller School of Medicine.)

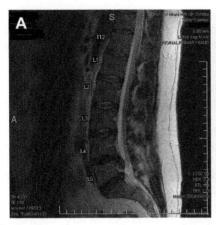
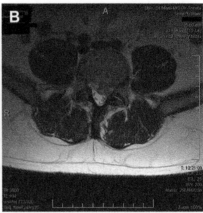

Fig. 5. (A) Lumbar magnetic resonance imaging (MRI), T2-weighted sagittal image. Note the disk extrusion with caudal migration at L4-5 disk. (B) Lumbar MRI, T2-weighted axial image from the same patient. Note the displacement of the left L5 nerve root. (*Courtesy of* the University of Miami- Miller School of Medicine.)

for larger herniated disks, extruded disks, and sequestered disks, which are less often seen in asymptomatic patients.

MRI increases the nonspinal incidental findings, including renal cysts, liver cysts, thyroid nodules, and lymph node enlargement. All these conditions have the potential to be malignant, so they often require follow-up testing. But malignancy is extremely rare with these findings, thus the burden of cost and care is increased. Recently, higher-resolution scanners with 3.0 tesla and even stronger magnets have been introduced. It remains to be seen if this introduction results in a greater ability to find abnormality or an increase in incidental findings and reduced specificity (**Figs. 9–13**).

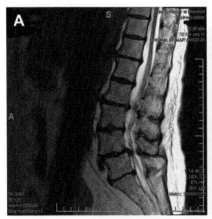
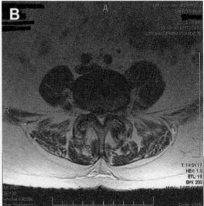

Fig. 6. (A) Lumbar magnetic resonance image (MRI), T2-weighted sagittal image. Note anterolisthesis of L4 on L5. (B) Lumbar MRI, T2-weighted axial image. Note severe bilateral facet/ligamentum flavum hypertrophy as well as prominence of the dorsal and bilateral ventral epidural fat, and a right paracentral disk protrusion, contributing to severe canal stenosis/thecal sac compression as well as severe left neural foraminal narrowing and mild to moderate right neural foraminal narrowing. Also note the prominent atrophy of the multifidus muscle. (*Courtesy of* the University of Miami- Miller School of Medicine.)

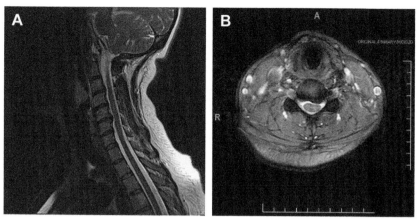

Fig. 7. (A) A C5-C6 disk herniation. (B) Left-sided C5-C6 disk protrusion. (*Courtesy of* the University of Miami- Miller School of Medicine.)

CT SCAN

Another imaging modality is the CT scan. CT scan gives a superior depiction of cortical bone than MRI and corrects the disadvantage of the latter that it cannot directly visualize cortical bone as well (although higher resolution scans are eliminating this problem).[3] CT scan can often better depict subtle fractures such as spondylolysis. CT scan is sometimes (not always) less expensive than MRI. CT scan can often see subtle foraminal abnormality much better than MRI, including bone spurs and lateral recess stenosis (**Figs. 15** and **16**). The final advantage of CT scan comes when the

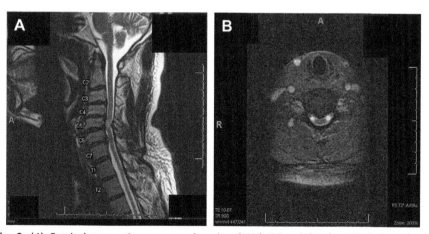

Fig. 8. (A) Cervical magnetic resonance imaging (MRI), T2-weighted sagittal view shows moderate to severe degenerative changes of the cervical spine greatest from C3-4 through C6-7 where prominent disk osteophyte complexes at C6-7 superimposed on right paracentral protrusion, contributing to pronounced canal stenosis with cord compression along these levels, most severe at C4-5 and C5-6. High T2 cord signal is noted along these levels, suggesting myelomalacia. (B) Cervical MRI, T2 axial view at the C6-7 level. (*Courtesy of* the University of Miami- Miller School of Medicine.)

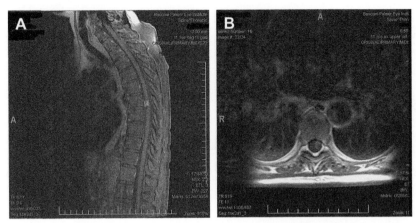

Fig. 9. (*A*) T1-weighted thoracic magnetic resonance image (MRI), sagittal view enhanced with gadolinium. The image shows thoracic meningioma at T6-7 causing radicular symptoms. (*B*) T1-weighted thoracic MRI, axial view enhanced with gadolinium. Note the enhancement in the thecal sac consistent with a meningioma. (*Courtesy of* the University of Miami- Miller School of Medicine.)

patient has a contraindication to have an MRI, such as a pacemaker, or metallic artifacts.

However, the disadvantages of CT scan in spinal imaging as a stand-alone study are significant. CT scan fails to show clearly soft tissue pathology such as disk material, nerve edema, spinal cord pathology, granulation tissue, infection, and inflammation

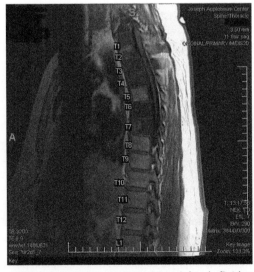

Fig. 10. Thoracic magnetic resonance image, T1-weighted fluid-attenuated inversion recovery sagittal image. The finding is consistent with parotid metastatic cancer of the vertebrae at multiple levels. (*Courtesy of* the University of Miami- Miller School of Medicine.)

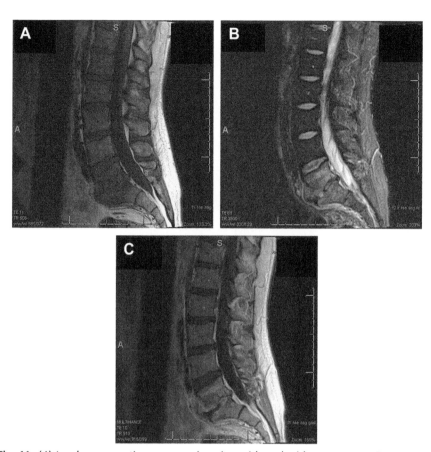

Fig. 11. (A) Lumbar magnetic resonance imaging with and without contrast. T1 sequence shows irregularity and enhancement of the inferior end plate of L5 and the superior end plate of S1 as well as the intervertebral disk space, consistent with discitis osteomyelitis. (B) T2 sequence. (C) T1 sequence after the administration of gadolinium. (*Courtesy of* the University of Miami- Miller School of Medicine.)

when compared with MRI. Although disk herniation can be visualized on the CT scan, the disk morphology cannot (see **Fig. 14**). Thus, findings of disk desiccation and annular tear often cannot be seen. The radiation exposure in a CT scan is also very high and should be considered when an MRI has a theoretical zero radiation exposure.

One way to enhance the CT scan is to add an intrathecal contrast (ie, as a myelogram). The procedure involves injecting an iodine-containing water-soluble contrast into the intrathecal space via a spinal injection. The contrast enhances the cerebrospinal fluid (CSF) delineating the thecal sac and the spinal nerves exiting the intervertebral foramen. CT myelography can therefore distinguish spinal nerves, spinal cord, and CSF. Thus, the compression of these neural structures can be identified. CT myelography can also sometimes better evaluate patients with surgical hardware, in whom MRI is nondiagnostic because of the presence of metal artifact, or those who have a contraindication to have an MRI. With the availability of MRI, which can adequately visualize the neural structures for most patients, especially advanced techniques in MRI, myelography has lost much of its popularity and utility.

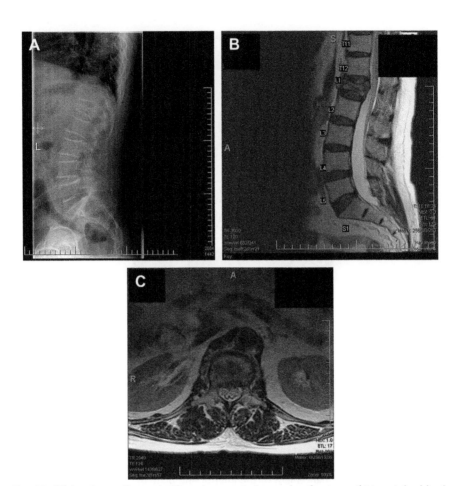

Fig. 12. (*A*) Lumbar radiograph. There is an anterior wedge fracture of L1 vertebral body with height loss of at least 50% at the anterior aspect. (*B*) Lumbar magnetic resonance image shows recent compression fracture of the L1 vertebra of the same patient. (*C*) Axial view retropulsion of bone into the spinal canal at the L1 level. (*Courtesy of* the University of Miami- Miller School of Medicine.)

CT scan and MRI were compared in a study by Thornbury and colleagues.[9] For herniated disks, CT scan had a sensitivity of 88% to 94% and a specificity of 57% to 64%, which was similar to the sensitivity and specificity of MRI. A meta-analysis of imaging tests for the diagnosis of stenosis[10] reported sensitivity ranging from 70% to 100% and specificity ranging from 80% to 96%. Other investigators found CT scan to accurately depict the foraminal and extraforaminal nerve root displacement or compression but confirmed that the CT scan is less effective for evaluating the intrathecal neurology.[11] The lateral recess can be narrowed because of many factors including osteophytes from facet/uncovertebral joints or vertebral bodies, herniated disks, or narrowed disks collapsing the foraminal size downward as well.[2]

Jarvik and Deyo[2] reported that the sensitivity and specificity of MRI for herniated disks were slightly higher than those for CT but similar for the diagnosis of spinal stenosis. They also concluded that advanced imaging should be reserved for patients

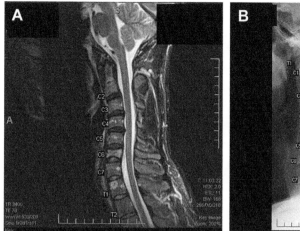
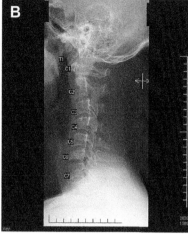

Fig. 13. (*A*) Cervical magnetic resonance image, sagittal T2 view. There is acute to subacute compression fracture at C6 with no significant retropulsion and no canal stenosis. (*B*) Cervical radiograph shows a fracture deformity of the vertebral body of C6 in the same patient. (*Courtesy of* the University of Miami- Miller School of Medicine.)

who are considering surgery or those in whom systemic disease is strongly suspected.[2]

SELECTIVE NERVE ROOT BLOCK

Selective nerve root block (SNRB) is a minimally invasive procedure that uses fluoroscopy. Fluoroscopy is real-time radiographic imaging that allows for dynamic

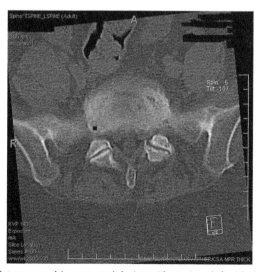

Fig. 14. Computed tomographic scan, axial view. There is a left-sided disk protrusion at L5-S1 abutting the descending left S1 nerve root. (*Courtesy of* the University of Miami-Miller School of Medicine.)

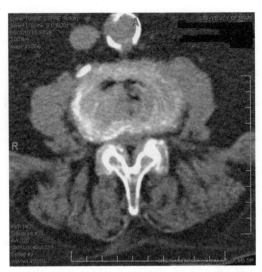

Fig. 15. Computed tomographic scan, axial view. Note the calcified disk bulge and the mild facet hypertrophy and ligamentum flavum thickening. There is moderate to severe canal stenosis. The neural foramina are mildly narrowed. (*Courtesy of* the University of Miami-Miller School of Medicine.)

assessment of the spine. This dynamic real-time ability allows for injection procedures to access specific foramen (nerve), bone, and joint structures in the spine. Such injections can be used to administer anesthetics to diagnose sources of pain from radiculopathy and other spinal pain in real-time (**Figs. 17** and **18**).

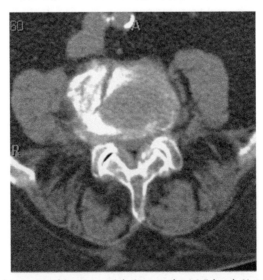

Fig. 16. Computed tomographic scan, axial view at the L4-5 level. Note that there is disk bulge, mild facet hypertrophy, and ligamentum flavum thickening. The right neural foramen is severely narrowed and it seems that the herniated disk compresses the right L4 nerve root as it exits the foramen. The left neural foramen also appears at least moderately stenosed. (*Courtesy of* the University of Miami- Miller School of Medicine.)

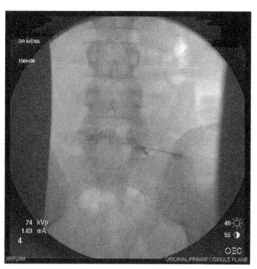

Fig. 17. A right L5 SNRB. (*Courtesy of* the University of Miami- Miller School of Medicine.)

By applying cortisone or other newly discovered drugs, such injections can also provide therapeutic benefit not available with other treatment techniques. In the case of radiculopathy, the intention of a transforaminal injection is to reduce inflammation around the spinal nerve and thereby decrease or relieve the pain.

When the needle is placed specifically low in the foramen in an extraepidural location, with low injection volume, more diagnostic information can be obtained on that specific spinal nerve. Too much epidural spread allows adjacent spinal nerves to be anesthetized and decrease the sensitivity of the diagnosis. Rubinstein and van Tulder[12] reviewed the literature and incorporated 9 studies that examined patients with radiculopathy. It was concluded that the sensitivity and specificity of an SNRB

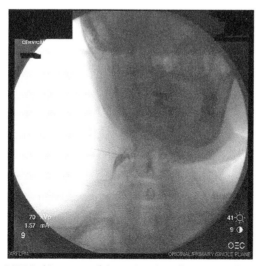

Fig. 18. A right C5-6 SNRB. (*Courtesy of* the University of Miami- Miller School of Medicine.)

ranged from 45% to 100% and that it may be an effective technique for evaluating patients with multilevel abnormality in order to ascertain the level of the pain generator.[12] Another systematic review examined the diagnostic accuracy of SNRBs for patients with radiculopathy and concluded that selective nerve root injections may be helpful as a diagnostic tool in evaluating spinal pain with radicular features. However, their role needs to be further clarified by additional research and consensus.[13]

Two studies reviewed patients with radicular pain in the cervical spine. One showed that there was a positive surgical response with a positive nerve-root block. In the second study, the investigators were interested in dermatomal mapping with SNRB. They found that referral patterns differed in some cases from the classic dermatomal maps. However, the investigators concluded that although SNRB may be helpful as a diagnostic tool, there is limited evidence of its effectiveness.[2]

BONE SCINTIGRAPHY

Bone scintigraphy is another method of identifying sites of bone disorder caused by altered metabolic activity.[14] This is considered another modality of choice for imaging the spine. Bone scintigraphy involves the administration of radioactive compounds that adhere to metabolically active bones.[2] Most commonly, these compounds are diphosphonate derivatives radiolabeled with technetium 99, which have a high affinity for bone and accumulate in areas of increased osteoblastic activity and blood flow.[2,15,16]

The main use of bone scintigraphy in spinal imaging is to investigate for (rule out) bony tumor such as metastasis, infection, or fractures, including insufficiency fractures. Each of these conditions show as a hyperintensity in the bone. The most common areas to look for insufficiency fractures are the sacrum and pars of the spine and the femoral neck of the hip, and for compression fractures, the vertebral bodies. Malignancies present with a typical pattern of hyperintensity, nonsymmetric, and can also be seen in areas outside the spine such as the ribs or pelvis because the bone scan surveys the entire skeleton. Because the bone scan shows hyperintensity in areas of osteoblastic activity, there may be no multiple myeloma because this is primarily a problem of pure osteoclastic lytic activity (unless there are pathologic fractures) (**Fig. 19**).

The main drawback of bone scintigraphy is that degenerative pathology usually will also show a positive result on the scan. This does not allow clear differentiation between degenerative changes in the spine caused by painful lesions and those caused by malignant lesions if the malignancy is early or low grade.[17] Bone scan is very sensitive in detecting abnormal joint loading, which leads to joint stress and eventual osteophyte formation by detecting abnormal uptake before any morphologic change appears.[13,15] This abnormal uptake may persist until the osteophyte shows maturation and there is stabilization of the arthritic bone. At this point, the uptake may decrease.[15,17–19] Often, with a fracture, infection, or high-grade malignancy, the level of hyperintensity is greater than that of degenerative changes. Also, degenerative abnormalities are more often present in and around the joints, where the malignancy or fracture can be more often midbone or in typical loading areas such as the femoral neck.

There are several scintigraphic techniques that might be useful for evaluating spinal conditions, including single photon emission CT (SPECT) and triple phase bone scans.

Triple phase bone scan is useful for diagnosing conditions, such as osteomyelitis,[2] and heterotopic ossification[20] involves the administration of a radioactive compound,

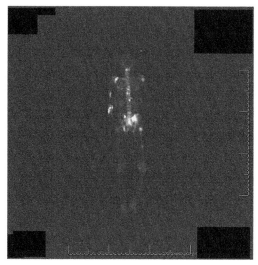

Fig. 19. Whole body scan shows multifocal increased osteoblastic activity in the patient with right C5-6 SNRB consistent with widespread metastatic disease to the bone skeleton as described. (*Courtesy of* the University of Miami- Miller School of Medicine.)

most commonly technetium 99m–labeled phosphate complexes, followed by imaging 2 to 4 hours after the administration. Three different images are taken, which includes dynamic flow and blood pool images for the diagnosis of inflammation and/or hyperemia along with the standard delayed images.[2]

SPECT is a scintigraphic technique for obtaining multiplanar views, using a rotating gamma camera.[14,18] SPECT has been widely used in patients with axial pain, especially for the diagnosis of zygapophyseal joint arthritis.[21] Several studies have shown that SPECT results correlate with response to injections to the zygapophyseal joints.[22–26] In these studies, the improvement after a zygapophyseal injection after correlating with an abnormal SPECT result ranges between 79% and 100%.[22,23,25,26] No study has correlated SPECT findings in the zygapophyseal joint to findings on MRI, such as facet hypertrophy or synovial swelling.

SUMMARY

Imaging studies to evaluate for radiculopathies should be used as an extension of the history and physical examination to confirm the suspected findings and exclude more serious and malignant pathologic conditions. Imaging can be used therapeutically to guide interventional procedures and help plan medical or surgical treatment. However, because of the high sensitivity of detecting abnormalities with questionable specificity, imaging studies should not be used in isolation or as a replacement of history taking and examination.

ACKNOWLEDGMENTS

The authors would like to thank Dr Ivan Castellon, MD, Neuroradiology fellow at the University of Miami Miller School of Medicine.

REFERENCES

1. van Tulder Maurits W, Assendelft W, Koes B, et al. Spinal radiographic findings and nonspecific low back pain: a systematic review of observational studies. Spine 1997;22:427–34.
2. Jarvik J, Deyo R. Diagnostic evaluation of low back pain with emphasis on imaging. Ann Intern Med 2002;137:586–95.
3. Lateef H, Patel P. What is the role of imaging in acute low back pain. Curr Rev Musculoskelet Med 2009;2:69–73.
4. Spitzer WO. Scientific approach to the assessment and management of activity-related spinal disorders: a monograph for clinicians. Report of the Quebec Task Force on Spinal Disorders. Spine 1987;12(7 Suppl):1–59.
5. Atlas S, Deyo R, Patrick D, et al. The Quebec Task Force classification for spinal disorders and the severity, treatment, and outcomes of sciatica and lumbar spinal stenosis. Spine 1996;21(24):2885–92.
6. Chou R, Qaseem A, Snow V, et al. Diagnosis and treatment of low back pain: a joint clinical practice guideline from the American College of Physicians and the American Pain Society. Ann Intern Med 2007;147(7):478–91.
7. Sheehan NJ. Magnetic resonance imaging for low back pain: indications and limitations. Ann Rheum Dis 2010;69:7–11.
8. Jensen M, Brant-Zawadzki M, Obuchowski N, et al. Magnetic resonance imaging of the lumbar spine in people without back pain. N Engl J Med 1994;331:69–73.
9. Thornbury JR, Fryback DG, Turski PA, et al. Disk-caused nerve compression in patients with acute low-back pain: diagnosis with MR, CT myelography, and plain CT. Radiology 1993;186:731–8.
10. Kent DL, Haynor DR, Larson EB, et al. Diagnosis of lumbar spinal stenosis in adults: a metaanalysis of the accuracy of CT, MR, and myelography. AJR Am J Roentgenol 1992;158:1135–44.
11. Wilmink JT. CT morphology of intrathecal lumbosacral nerve-root compression. AJNR Am J Neuroradiol 1989;10:233–48.
12. Rubinstein SM, van Tulder M. A best-evidence review of diagnostic procedures for neck and low-back pain [review]. Best Pract Res Clin Rheumatol 2008;22(3):471–82.
13. Everett CR, Shah RV, Sehgal N, et al. A systematic review of diagnostic utility of selective nerve root blocks. Pain Physician 2005;8(2):225–33.
14. Ryan RJ, Gibson T, Fogelman I. The identification of spinal pathology in chronic low back pain using single photon emission computed tomography. Nucl Med Commun 1992;13:497–502.
15. Omoumi P, Mercier GA, Lecouvet F, et al. CT arthrography, MR arthrography, PET, and scintigraphy in osteoarthritis. Radiol Clin North Am 2009;47:595–615.
16. McKillop JH, Fogelman I. Bone scintigraphy in benign bone disease. Br Med J (Clin Res Ed) 1984;288:264–6.
17. O'Neill C, Owens D. Role of single photon emission computed tomography in the diagnosis of chronic low back pain. Spine J 2010;10:70–2.
18. Merrick MV. Investigation of joint disease. Eur J Nucl Med 1992;19:894–901.
19. Kim KY, Wang MY. Magnetic resonance image-based morphological predictors of single photon emission computed tomography-positive facet arthropathy in patients with axial back pain. Neurosurgery 2006;59:147–56.
20. Shehab D, Elgazzar AH, Collier BD. Heterotopic ossification. J Nucl Med 2002;43(3):346–53.

21. Makki D, Khazim R, Zaidan A, et al. Single photon emission computerized tomography (SPECT) scan-positive facet joints and other spinal structures in a hospital-wide population with spinal pain. Spine J 2010;10(1):58–62.
22. Holder L, Marchin J, Asdourian P, et al. Planar and high resolution SPECT bone imaging in the diagnosis of facet syndrome. J Nucl Med 1995;36:37–44.
23. Dolan A, Ryan P, Arden N, et al. The value of SPECT scans in identifying back pain likely to benefit from facet joint injection. Br J Rheumatol 1996;35:1269–73.
24. Ackerman W, Ahmad M. Pain relief with intraarticular or medial branch nerve blocks in patients with positive lumbar facet joint SPECT imaging: a 12-week outcome study. South Med J 2008;101:931–4.
25. McDonald M, Cooper R, Wang M. Use of computed tomography-single-photon emission computed tomography fusion for diagnosing painful facet arthropathy technical note. Neurosurg Focus 2007;22:E2.
26. Pneumaticos S, Chatziioannou S, Hipp J, et al. Low back pain: prediction of short-term outcome of facet joint injection with bone scintigraphy. Radiology 2006;238:693–8.

The Electrodiagnostic Evaluation of Radiculopathy

Christopher T. Plastaras, MD*, Anand B. Joshi, MD, MHA

KEYWORDS

• Electromyography • Radiculopathy • Electrodiagnosis
• Spinal stenosis

The clinical diagnosis of radiculitis indicates limb pain emanating from a spinal nerve or spinal nerve root. Objective findings of strength or reflex deficits or electrodiagnostic changes suggest nerve root dysfunction termed *radiculopathy*. Although commonly caused by structural lesions, such a herniated nucleus pulposus or degenerative spondylosis, radiculopathy can also be caused by inflammatory, infectious, or malignant disorders.[1] Structural causes of radiculopathy may be readily apparent through common imaging modalities, such as MRI or computed axial tomography.[2] However, MRI is associated with a significantly high false-positive rate in asymptomatic individuals and increases with age.[3,4] In such equivocal cases, imaging may be complemented by electrodiagnostic testing. Electrodiagnostic testing is a functional evaluation of the nervous system. Electrodiagnostic testing also has the added benefit of allowing objective documentation of the chronicity and severity of peripheral nervous system disease.[5]

DEFINITION

Electrodiagnosis is a broad term encompassing multiple electrodiagnostic techniques, including needle electrode examination (NEE); motor and sensory nerve conduction studies (NCS), including late responses; and evoked potentials. These tests are frequently used in various combinations in the evaluation of radiculopathy primarily to rule out other disorders in the peripheral and central nervous system; however, the NEE is considered the crucial component in the electrodiagnostic evaluation of radiculopathy. To meet the electrodiagnostic criteria for a radiculopathy, abnormalities must be demonstrated in at least 2 muscles innervated by the same nerve root but different peripheral nerves with no abnormalities detected in muscles innervated by the adjacent nerve roots.

The authors have nothing to disclose.
Penn Spine Center, Department of Physical Medicine & Rehabilitation, University of Pennsylvania, 3400 Spruce Street, Ground Floor, White Building, Philadelphia, PA 19104, USA
* Corresponding author.
E-mail address: Christopher.plastaras@uphs.upenn.edu

Phys Med Rehabil Clin N Am 22 (2011) 59–74
doi:10.1016/j.pmr.2010.10.005
1047-9651/11/$ – see front matter © 2011 Elsevier Inc. All rights reserved.

HISTORY AND EXAMINATION

The symptoms of many musculoskeletal and peripheral nerve disorders overlap with the clinical presentation of radiculopathy, therefore electrodiagnostic testing may be ordered for these populations to aide in establishing a diagnosis. Electrodiagnostic testing is not infallible and may be painful and expensive, therefore, as with many other forms of advanced diagnostic testing, electrodiagnosis should only be used as an extension of the history and physical examination. There have been studies done to evaluate the relationship between physical examination and electrodiagnostics. When 170 subjects were referred to an electrodiagnostic laboratory, 32% were diagnosed with a musculoskeletal disorder by standardized physical examination.[6] However, of those subjects with normal electrodiagnostic studies, the prevalence of musculoskeletal disorders increased to 55%. When there was electrodiagnostic evidence of radiculopathy, the presence of a musculoskeletal disorder was still 21%. The significant overlap between the presence of lower-extremity musculoskeletal disorders and lumbosacral radiculopathy suggests that the presence or absence of a musculoskeletal diagnosis does not accurately predict which patients will have normal electrodiagnostic studies.[6] In another study Lauder and colleagues[7] calculated sensitivities, specificities, and predictive values of various symptoms and signs for those with an abnormal electrodiagnostic study. No historical feature was found to be significantly associated with an abnormal electrodiagnostic study. The most sensitive historical feature was the presence of radicular leg pain (86%), though this symptom had a specificity of only 12%. The investigators evaluated several physical examination findings and found the following sensitivities and specificities (sensitivity/specificity): reduced vibration or pinprick sensation (50%/62%), Achilles or patellar reflex deficit (25%/87%), weakness of any muscle (69%/53%), and positive straight leg raise (21%/87%). However, in subjects that had any 4 abnormal physical findings there was a greater than 6 times likelihood that the electromyogram (EMG) study would be abnormal when compared with cases with a normal physical examination.

As with lumbosacral radiculopathies, the value of the history and physical examination in predicting cervical radiculopathies has also been studied.[8] Subjects with symptoms of numbness, tingling, and subjective weakness were more than twice as likely to have abnormal electrodiagnostic testing.[8] Unfortunately, none of these symptoms were significant for radiculopathy specifically. In contrast, the presence of weakness, abnormal reflexes, or abnormal sensation on physical examination indicates a greater than 4 times likelihood of having an abnormal electrodiagnostic study, with a greater than 2 times likelihood of confirming a cervical radiculopathy. A particularly valuable physical examination finding is an abnormal biceps reflex, which increases the odds ratio of making an EMG diagnosis of cervical radiculopathy to 10. In general, the combination of having weakness and a reduced reflex was a strong predictor of both an abnormal electrodiagnostic study, including radiculopathy specifically. Notably, up to 48% of individuals with abnormal electrodiagnostic results will have a normal physical examination, emphasizing the physical examination's relative lack of sensitivity when using electrodiagnosis as a gold standard.

NERVE ROOT VARIATION

As previously described, the electrodiagnosis of radiculopathy relies upon a myotomal pattern of abnormalities found on NEE. However, variation in the anatomic pattern of nerve roots is known to exist and must be accounted for in the interpretation of the NEE. A study of 200 spontaneously aborted fetuses revealed 107 (53.5%) to show significant variation from the most common arrangement of the brachial plexus.[9]

The most common variants of brachial plexus organization are described as the *prefixed* and *postfixed* plexus. These variants have been variously defined[10] and emphasize the contributions of the C4 and T2 roots. A prefixed plexus is characterized by a C4 branch that is larger than the branch from T2.[11] The electromyographic implications of this are that C4 may contribute to the innervation of the shoulder girdle musculature, which is more typically C5. In contrast, a postfixed plexus contains a large contribution from T2, and a small contribution from C4.[11] Prefixation may be seen in up to 48% of specimens[9,12]; whereas, postfixation is seen in 0.5% to 4.0% of cases.[9,12]

Precise localization through the NEE is similarly challenged in the electrodiagnosis of lumbosacral radiculopathy. Though the vast majority of lumbosacral radiculopathies occur at either L5 (47.6%) or S1 (30%),[13] both of these nerve roots may show significant variation from normal patterns of innervations. In a study of 50 subjects undergoing lumbar decompression surgery, intraoperative stimulation of the L5 and S1 nerve roots revealed 16% to have significant deviations from normal.[14] Common anomalies in this study include dominant nerve roots that were expressed more heavily in muscles than normal, and such anomalies were more frequent in subjects with transitional vertebral segments. A novel study[15] compared the neurologic symptoms generated by selective nerve root blocks using electrical stimulation in subjects with transitional and normal lumbar segments. In this study, when L5 is sacralized, the function of the L5 nerve root becomes similar to the S1 nerve root. Such normal variations in peripheral nervous system anatomy must be accounted for in the performance of the NEE.

SENSITIVITY OF EMG

Although the diagnosis of radiculopathy hinges upon the NEE, the sensitivity of EMG in detecting radiculopathy is limited by several factors. First this procedure is targeted exclusively toward motor axons. Radiculopathies with predominant sensory root involvement, even if severe, will not elicit any needle electrode abnormalities.[5] However, substantial demyelinating disease may be detected on the NEE by changes in motor unit recruitment. Unfortunately, significant demyelination at the level of the nerve root is uncommon.[5] Secondly, the electrodiagnostic confirmation of a radiculopathy rests upon an identification of a myotomal pattern of abnormalities. Such identification may not occur if axonal compromise is not severe enough to be detected by the needle electrode or widespread enough to localize to a particular myotome.[16] Thirdly, the appearance of fibrillation potentials is time dependent and may not appear in limb muscles several weeks after axonal damage.[16] Therefore, if done too early, an NEE will not appreciate fibrillations because they have not yet developed. Also, if done too late, fibrillation potentials are known to shrink because of muscle atrophy and thus become more difficult to appreciate. This effect has happened 6 months after the onset of cervical radiculopathies[17] and 12 to 18 months after the onset of lumbosacral radiculopathies.[5]

Besides these inherent limitations, measurement of the sensitivity of electrodiagnostic studies is complicated by the lack of a gold standard. In determining the sensitivity of electrodiagnostic testing, various criterion standards have been used, such as clinical, surgical, and radiological findings. The clinical sensitivity of electrodiagnostic testing in lumbosacral radiculopathy ranges between 49%[18] and 84%.[14] Haig and colleagues[19] performed a stringent study using validated, anatomic needle placement into the limb muscles and a quantified "paraspinal mapping" technique to evaluate the sensitivity and specificity of electrodiagnostic testing in lumbar spinal stenosis. The composite limb and paraspinal fibrillation score showed a sensitivity of 47.8% and a specificity of 87.5%. This finding agrees with the 44% sensitivity and 86% specificity obtained by Coster and colleagues[20] using radiological evidence of nerve root compression as a gold standard. In comparison, although the prevalence of both disc bulges and protrusions increases with age, if not stratified by age, MRI of the lumbar spine shows a specificity of 36%; only 36% of people without back pain will have a normal disc at all levels.[4] The much higher sensitivity of MRI justifies its appropriateness as a screening test; whereas, the greater specificity of electrodiagnostics suggests that it is better used as a confirmatory test.

Similar to lumbosacral radiculopathy, the electrodiagnostic evaluation of cervical radiculopathies also shows a wide range of sensitivities, from 50%[21] to 95%.[22] The false positive rate of cervical MRI is somewhat lower, but still significant at 14% of asymptomatic individuals aged less than 40 years and 28% of those aged greater than 40 years.[3] Therefore, electrodiagnostics and MRI can be complementary rather than competing modalities. Electrodiagnostic studies and MRI will agree in 60% of patients with symptoms suggestive of radiculopathy and in 76% of cases when weakness is present.[2]

SENSORY NERVE CONDUCTION STUDIES

Abnormalities in sensory nerve action potentials (SNAP) are not part of the electrodiagnostic criteria of radiculopathy. However, their performance is necessary to evaluate for other disorders that are part of the differential diagnosis of radiculopathy, such as peripheral polyneuropathy or entrapment mononeuropathy.[23] As symptoms of pain are typically mediated by C-fibers, which are too small to be accessible by standard electrodiagnostic techniques, sensory nerve parameters, such as amplitude, distal latency, and nerve conduction velocity, are not expected to be abnormal in radiculopathy.[24] Also, in radiculopathy the usual location of the lesion is proximal to the dorsal root ganglion, and degeneration will proceed centrally rather than peripherally.[5] However, important exceptions to this dictum must be recognized. When pathology extends from the intraspinal space into the neural foramen and affects the dorsal root ganglion, as can happen with malignancy or infection, SNAP amplitude reduction will occur as a result of wallerian degeneration.[24] Additionally, SNAP amplitudes may be reduced when the dorsal root ganglion has an intraspinal location making it vulnerable to lesions resulting from lumbar spondylosis. This reduction may occur in L5 radiculopathies, causing reduction of superficial peroneal nerve amplitudes. Reduction of superficial peroneal nerve amplitudes are seen in 21.1% of patients with L5 radiculopathy who are aged less than 60 years.[25]

Evaluation of possible entrapment mononeuropathy is an important reason to perform nerve conduction studies in the electrodiagnostic evaluation of radiculopathy. For example, the prevalence of carpal tunnel syndrome in patients with cervical radiculopathy has been estimated at 22.1%,[26] which is significantly greater than estimates for the general population (0.52% for men and 1.49% for women).[27] The double crush hypothesis was put forth in 1973 by Upton and McComas and proposes that a proximal lesion along an axon, such as that caused by radiculopathy, predisposes it to injury at a more distal site.[28] Such a mechanism is one hypothesis as to why the incidence of carpal tunnel syndrome seems to be increased in patients with cervical radiculopathy.[26] However, another study did not reveal any correlation between the presence of C6 or C7 radiculopathy and abnormal median sensory responses and C8 radiculopathy and abnormal median motor responses.[29] Prior studies have shown similar results.[30,31] Other possible reasons why the incidence of carpal tunnel syndrome is increased in patients with cervical radiculopathy is that both disorders have a common etiology, such as osteoarthritis that leads to both cervical foraminal and carpal tunnel stenosis.[26]

MOTOR NERVE CONDUCTION STUDIES

Compound muscle action potentials (CMAP) may be abnormal in the presence of a radiculopathy if axon loss is occurring. The amplitude of the CMAP can provide a semiquantitative measure of the number of axons supplying the muscle from which the recording was made.[32] Therefore, L5 and S1 radiculopathies may cause reduction of peroneal CMAPs, recording from the extensor digitorum brevis and the abductor hallucis, respectively. However, the CMAP amplitude is not perfectly sensitive to the presence of a lumbosacral radiculopathy. Significant reduction in CMAP amplitudes occurs with loss of approximately 50% of motor axons[24] and it is rare for this many nerve root fibers to degenerate.[5] Additionally, muscles typically have an overlapping nerve supply, allowing for redundancy even if individual nerve roots are compromised.

Another limitation of using the CMAP amplitude to diagnose is emphasized in the evaluation of cervical radiculopathies. The most commonly performed upper extremity motor nerve conduction studies are the median and ulnar motor nerve conduction studies to the abductor pollicis brevis and the abductor digiti minimi, respectively. These muscles are predominantly subserved by the C8 and T1 nerve roots. However, the most common cervical radiculopathies occur at C7 and C6,[5,33] implying that the most commonly performed upper extremity motor nerve conduction studies will be insensitive for the most common cervical radiculopathies.

LATE RESPONSES

Late responses are so named because their latency exceeds that of the more commonly studied M-wave. Their theoretical advantages include their ability to study the proximal nerve segments where the pathology of radiculopathy lies.

H Reflex

The H reflex was first described by Hoffman in 1918[34] and subsequently hypothesized by Magladery to be a monosynaptic reflex that assesses the afferent Ia sensory nerve and an efferent alpha motor nerve.[35] However, other experimental studies have concluded that the pathways generating the H reflex likely receive an oligosynaptic contribution.[36] In clinical practice, the H reflex is most commonly obtained by stimulating the tibial nerve in the popliteal fossa and recording over the gastroc-soleus to assess the S1 nerve root, although the H reflex may also be obtained from the flexor carpi radialis in the forearm. The H reflex requires a longer-duration stimulus that is optimally between 0.5 and 1.0 ms.[37] The sensitivity of the H reflex for nerve pathology has been estimated to be between 82%[38] and 89%,[39] and can be compromised through preferential sparing of the fibers that mediate the reflex.[5] However, specificity for radiculopathy is compromised by several factors. The entire H reflex arc travels through peripheral nerve, lumbosacral plexus, and spinal nerve roots. Abnormalities in any of these segments can disturb the H reflex[5] and cannot be considered specific for radiculopathy. Additionally, H reflexes may not normalize once they become abnormal, limiting their use in monitoring patients with known S1 radiculopathies.[5] Finally, H reflexes may be abnormal bilaterally in patients aged more than 60 years or secondary to peripheral polyneuropathy.[5] Both latency and amplitude have been used as parameters to evaluate the H reflex. Amplitude has been criticized as less sensitive[40] because of its variation with posture, muscle contracture, age, and temperature.[41] However, comparative studies have suggested amplitude ratio to be a better parameter of S1 radiculopathy, particularly when H reflexes are present bilaterally.[41] Various techniques have been described for eliciting the tibial H reflex (**Figs. 1** and **2**).[42,43]

More recently, a simple and reproducible method known as the *half and half* technique[44] described by Nishida has the advantages of producing a biphasic waveform with initial negative deflection. Such a waveform has easier-to-determine amplitude and latency parameters in comparison to the triphasic waveforms generated by the other methods (**Figs. 3** and **4**).[44] However, this method has no published normative data and has been criticized as producing nonphysiologic wave-forms; further study will be needed to determine its validity.[45]

The H reflex may also be obtained in the upper limb by recording from the flexor carpi radialis (FCR).[46] The H reflex may be obtained from the flexor carpi radialis in 90%[46] to 95%[47] of patients. This test may be used in the electrodiagnosis of C6 and C7 radiculopathies and will remain normal in patients with C5 and C8 radiculopathies.[48] The sensitivities and specificities of the FCR H-reflex have been found to be 50% and 86% for C6 radiculopathy and 75% and 86% for C7 radiculopathy.[49] The upper limit of normal latency is 21.0 ms with 1.5 ms of side-to-side variation.[34] The FCR H reflex may be elicited by the technique described by Jabre in which the E-1 is placed over the belly of the FCR (one-third of the distance between the medial epicondyle and radial styloid), the reference over the brachioradialis, and the ground between the stimulator and the E-1 electrode (**Figs. 5** and **6**)[46]:

F Wave

So named because they were originally recorded in the intrinsic foot muscles,[35] the F wave is a late response produced by supramaximal stimulation resulting in antidromic activation of motor neurons.[34] Latency is the parameter most frequently used in the evaluation of F waves.[34] Minimum latency is reported most commonly[24] but mean F wave latencies may dilute measurement error and produce more consistent results.[50] When used to evaluate L5/S1 radiculopathy, the sensitivity of F wave abnormalities is impressively close to that of the NEE.[51,52] Additionally, the F wave may be used as a dynamic test because standing for 3 minutes increases F-wave chronodispersion in patients with lumbar spinal stenosis.[53] However, the specificity of F waves may be limited by the dilution effect of latency abnormalities being hidden by the lengthy course of nerve fibers and, like H reflexes, abnormalities will result from any pathology affecting proximal nerve segments in addition to radiculopathy.[5]

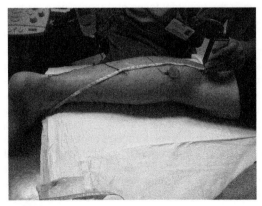

Fig. 1. Tibial H-Reflex Setup. (Technique suggested by Johnson and Braddom).

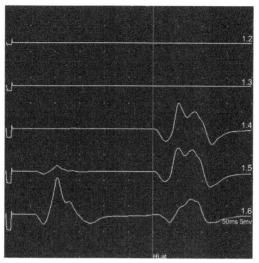

Fig. 2. Tibial H-Reflex Waveform. (Technique suggested by Johnson and Braddom).

EVOKED POTENTIALS

Evoked potentials are the responses of the central nervous system to external stimuli and somatosensory evoked potentials (SEP) occur as a result of stimulation of afferent peripheral nerve fibers.[54] The use of SEPs in the evaluation of radiculopathy remains controversial[16] and the most recent American Association of Neuromuscular and

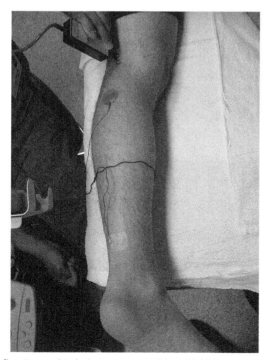

Fig. 3. Tibial H-Reflex Setup. (Technique suggested by Nishida).

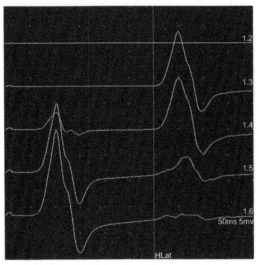

Fig. 4. Tibial H-Reflex Waveform. (Technique suggested by Nishida).

Electrodiagnostic Medicine (AANEM) guideline devoted to the subject indicated that dermatomal and sensory evoked potentials may be useful to direct further evaluation and treatment of lumbosacral spinal stenosis.[54] The great strength of dermatomal SEPs is their ability to evaluate segmental level function throughout the neuraxis, in contrast to mixed nerve action potential.[55] Kraft postulates that the abnormalities of lumbosacral spinal stenosis may be caused by demyelination caused by chronic compression,[55,56] rather than axon loss. Therefore, needle electrode examination may be unrevealing; whereas, conduction deficits may be readily detected by dermatomal SEPs. When using either computed tomography or MRI as a gold standard, dermatomal somatosensory evoked potentials are found to have 78% sensitivity and a 93% positive predictive value of multiple root disease indicative of spinal stenosis.[57]

However, somatosensory evoked potentials must be interpreted in light of their several disadvantages.[24] Dermatomal SEPs cannot distinguish between the various causes of multiple-root disease, such as lumbosacral spinal stenosis or arachnoiditis, and are also not felt to be useful for acute radiculopathy.[55,56,58] Amplitude

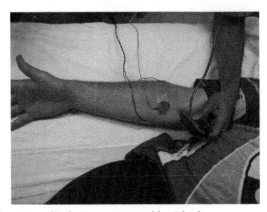

Fig. 5. FCR H-Reflex Setup. (Technique suggested by Jabre).

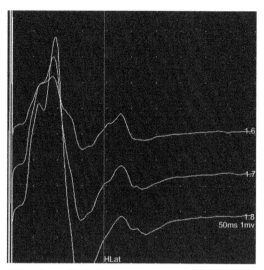

Fig. 6. FCR H-Reflex Waveform. (Technique suggested by Jabre).

measurements have too much normal variation to have clinical significance. Additionally, focal slowing in the root may be diluted by normal conduction in the remainder of the sensory pathway. Furthermore, somatosensory evoked potentials evaluate the larger fiber tracts modulating proprioception and vibration, rather than the pain-mediating tracts that seem to most commonly elicit symptoms. Finally, the technically demanding nature of the procedure combines with the previous limitations to discourage their routine use.[24]

NEEDLE ELECTRODE EXAMINATION

The concept of using a myotomal distribution of abnormalities on NEE to localize a spinal segment dates back to at least 1944[59] and is now a cornerstone of the electrodiagnosis of radiculopathy. The NEE is considered diagnostic of radiculopathy when abnormalities are noted in at least 2 muscles innervated by the same root, but different peripheral nerves, provided that muscles innervated by adjacent roots are normal.[5] Needle electromyography evaluates for axonal loss and will reveal demyelination through reduced recruitment of motor units only when conduction block is present.[5,24,60]

The NEE may also provide information regarding the length of time that a muscle has been denervated. A study of 69 subjects who suffered traumatic peripheral nerve injury revealed that fibrillation amplitude may be used as an index of estimating the time since nerve injury.[61] The mean amplitude of fibrillations within 2 months after denervation was 612 µV and decreased to less than 100 µV after 12 months. The same study found that reduction of fibrillation potential amplitudes also correlated with muscle fiber atrophy in a guinea pig model.[61]

Similar findings were replicated in the upper extremities of 173 subjects who suffered complete denervation of the biceps brachii caused by brachial plexus injury.[62] In this study, fibrillation amplitude within 2 months was 501 µV, but in contrast to Kraft's study, remained greater than 100 µV (262 µV) after 12 months. Consistent with prior animal studies,[61] the reduction in fibrillation amplitude correlated with muscle fiber atrophy and that Type II muscle fiber atrophy is more rapid than Type I.

The most recent AANEM guidelines indicate that, at least, one muscle in myotomes C5-T1 and cervical paraspinal muscles should be studied in the evaluation of cervical radiculopathy.[23] However, the guidelines do not specify how many muscles to study. Clearly, the NEE is uncomfortable to patients and studying the minimum number of muscles that is required is desirable. Additionally, not all radiculopathies are confirmable by EMG.[5] These radiculopathies are exclusively sensory[5] or radiculopathies in which the rate of denervation is balanced by the rate of reinnervation.[63] Radiculopathies that are not confirmable by EMG will not be found regardless of how many muscles are studied.[63] The concept of a screening NEE was developed to determine the minimum number of muscles that need to be studied to maximize the probability of detecting an electrodiagnostically confirmable radiculopathy.[63] A previous retrospective study[64] determined that 7-muscle screens that included cervical paraspinals would identify 93% to 98% of all electrodiagnostically confirmed cervical radiculopathies. However, prospective evidence specifying the optimal number of muscles to include in the NEE to detect a cervical radiculopathy arrived in 2001, when Dillingham and colleagues[65] determined that 6 muscles that included the cervical paraspinals was the optimal screen. When using motor recruitment changes as diagnostic criteria, a 6-muscle screen was found to identify 94% to 99% of cervical radiculopathies, with additional muscles adding only minimal sensitivity. An important point noted is that if paraspinal muscles cannot be studied, then 8-limb muscles are necessary to detect greater than 92% of cervical radiculopathies. Also notable is that the study does not prescribe a specific set of muscles, but rather indicates the number of muscles that must be studied. However, their data does indicate that various possible screens have differing specificities and sensitivities. For example, a screen of paraspinals, deltoid, triceps, pronator teres, extensor digitorum communis, and abductor pollicis brevis yielded sensitivity of 99% using recruitment changes as diagnostic and 83% using abnormal spontaneous activity as diagnostic.[65]

Finally, should any muscle be abnormal within the 6-muscle screen, additional muscles may need to be studied to confirm the radiculopathy.[65]

Similar to cervical radiculopathies, the optimal number of muscles required in the screening NEE of the lower extremities was not clearly elucidated until recently. Prior retrospective evidence[66] suggested that a 5-muscle screen was sufficient. However, subsequent evidence confirmed that, in fact, 6 muscles constitute the optimal screening NEE when paraspinals are included, and that 8 are required if paraspinals cannot be included.[63] As with cervical screening examinations, no specific combination of muscles is recommended, although varying sensitivities are clearly achieved with different muscles studied. For example, a screen of paraspinals, adductor longus, medial gastrocnemius, tibialis posterior, tibialis anterior, and short head biceps femoris yielded sensitivity of 100% using recruitment changes as diagnostic and 93% using abnormal spontaneous activity as diagnostic.[63] Even a 4-muscle screen that includes the paraspinals will detect 97% of lumbosacral radiculopathies.[63] Clearly, the screening NEE does not replace a directed history and physical examination. Rather, a screen provides a ceiling to the number of muscles studied when neither the history nor the physical examination are localizing and allow the NEE to be targeted toward specific abnormalities.[63–66]

A myotomal pattern of abnormalities on NEE is necessary for the diagnosis of radiculopathy. These abnormalities may encompass any of a variety of neuropathic findings, such as polyphasia, reduced recruitment, increased insertional activity, complex repetitive discharges, or large-amplitude and long-duration motor unit action potentials (MUAP). With chronic denervation and subsequent reinnervation, the duration of MUAPs increases, commensurate with the degree of collateral sprouting.[5,16] Unfortunately, reliably determining MUAP duration requires the quantitative evaluation of at least 20 motor units,[67] which is far too lengthy a procedure to recommend for clinical practice. Polyphasic MUAPs contain greater than 4 phases and may indicate motor unit remodeling caused by chronic denervation and reinnervation.[5,16] Early series[68,69] indicated that isolated polyphasia may be the only finding in 35% to 75% of cases. However, using polyphasia as the sole diagnostic criterion for radiculopathy is problematic. Polyphasic MUAPs are not inherently abnormal and up to 20% of MUAPs in normal muscle may be polyphasic.[5,16] As with duration, differentiation of true polyphasia from pseudopolyphasia requires the use of a delay and trigger line,[70] which may not be done in routine NEE.

The use of spontaneous activity, such as fibrillations and positive sharp waves, may be more reliable than the motor unit remodeling parameters previously described. However, certain pitfalls must also be recognized with these. Conventionally, spontaneous activity occurring after acute radiculopathy is thought to appear first in the paraspinals in approximately 1 week and to manifest in more distal limb muscles in several weeks,[5,16] indicating that an improperly timed study may miss abnormalities. However, recent prospective evidence has challenged this long-held theory, and indicated no correlation between the presence of paraspinal spontaneous activity and symptom duration in both the cervical and lumbar spine.[71]

SEGMENTAL LOCALIZATION

In 50 subjects with surgically proven single-root lesions, the following patterns of positive sharp waves or fibrillations on NEE emerged[72]:

- C5 radiculopathy: In C5 radiculopathy, the infraspinatus, supraspinatus, biceps, deltoid, and brachioradialis showed approximately equal incidences of spontaneous activity.
- C6 radiculopathy: A C6 root lesion produces the most variable pattern of abnormalities and can mimic the findings of C5 radiculopathy with the addition of pronator teres and the other pattern quite similar to that of a C7 radiculopathy.
- C7 radiculopathy: In C7 radiculopathies, the flexor carpi radialis, anconeus, pronator teres, and triceps were most frequently affected.
- C8 radiculopathy: C8 radiculopathy most typically affected the first dorsal interosseus; extensor indicus proprius; abductor digiti minimi; and, less frequently, the flexor pollicis longus and abductor pollicis brevis.[72]

A similar study was conducted of the preoperative needle electrode patterns of 45 subjects with surgically documented single-level lumbosacral radiculopathies and showed the following[38]:

- L2-4: No meaningful pattern was found that distinguished one level from another. This finding may be because of the low incidence of radiculopathies at these levels (7 subjects). This finding correlates with previous estimates of only 10% of lumbosacral radiculopathies affecting these nerve roots.[70] Surprisingly, none of the confirmed L4 radiculopathies in this series showed involvement of the tibialis anterior.
- L5: The muscles affected most of the time (73%–100%) were peroneus longus, tensor fascia lata, tibialis posterior, extensor digitorum brevis, tibialis anterior, and extensor hallucis longus. However, needle electrode localization of the peroneus longus may be inaccurate, perhaps reducing the value of studying this muscle.[73]
- S1: The muscles affected most of the time (64%–100%) were the long head of the biceps femoris, lateral gastrocnemius, short head of the biceps femoris, medial gastrocnemius, abductor digiti quinti, and gluteus maximus.[38]

THE PARASPINAL MUSCLES

Abnormalities of the paraspinal muscles are considered to localize a lesion as being proximal to the plexus.[74] However, spontaneous activity in the paraspinals may be found in a variety of conditions, including diabetes[5]; after minor trauma, such as lumbar puncture[75]; after laminectomy[76]; and in up to 4% of asymptomatic, healthy people.[77] Notably, the presence of paraspinal abnormalities on needle electrode is not part of the electrodiagnostic criteria of radiculopathy.[23] Therefore, the evaluation of paraspinal abnormalities must be made in light of the remainder of the electrodiagnostic findings and in corroboration with the history and physical examination.

OUTCOMES

Electrodiagnosis may also be used as a prognostic indicator of epidural injections. A retrospective comparison has been conducted of 18 subjects with electrodiagnostically proven lumbosacral radiculopathy to 21 subjects with negative examinations,[78] all of whom underwent transforaminal epidural steroid injection (TFESI). Although the two groups had statistically similar preinjection Oswestry Disability Index (ODI) scores, the group with electrodiagnostically proven radiculopathy had significantly greater improvements in ODI scores after TFESI. The group with electrodiagnostic radiculopathy had higher, although statistically nonsignificant, scores upon the Verbal Rating Scales (VRS) of current pain. However, the improvement in mean VRS scores was not significantly different between the two groups following TFESI. The results of this study suggest that electrodiagnosis may serve an important prognostic function in guiding interventional spine procedures and that patients with electrodiagnostically proven radiculopathy may show significant functional improvements after TFESI.

Additionally, electrodiagnostic confirmation of a radiculopathy may have important implications when surgery is contemplated. In a small sample size study, Alrawi and colleagues[79] demonstrated that subjects with electrodiagnostically confirmed cervical radiculopathy had improved outcomes following discectomy and anterior fusion when compared with postoperative subjects who did not have electrophysiologic evidence of radiculopathy. Conversely, Tullberg and colleagues[80] studied 30 subjects with lumbosacral radiculopathy and demonstrated that when visual analogue scores were used as an outcome measure, the absence of electrodiagnostic confirmation was correlated with poor post-operative results.

SUMMARY

Radiculopathy is a sometimes challenging diagnosis resulting from multiple etiologies. Although imaging may elucidate the structural causes of radiculopathy, imaging cannot pinpoint the cause of radiculopathy when either multiple structural abnormalities are present or when radiculopathy results from nonstructural causes. Electrodiagnosis provides a means of functional assessment of the nerve root and may also provide prognostic information regarding functional outcomes of patients with radiculopathy.

REFERENCES

1. Shelerud RA, Paynter KS. Rarer causes of radiculopathy: spinal tumors, infections, and other unusual causes. Phys Med Rehabil Clin N Am 2002;13(3):645–96.
2. Nardin RA, Patel MR, Gudas TF, et al. Electromyography and magnetic resonance imaging in the evaluation of radiculopathy. Muscle Nerve 1999;22:151–5.

3. Boden SD, McCowin PR, Davis DO, et al. Abnormal magnetic-resonance scans of the cervical spine in asymptomatic subjects. J Bone Joint Surg Am 1990;72:1178–84.
4. Jensen MC, Brant-Zawadzki MN, Obuchowski N, et al. Magnetic resonance imaging of the lumbar spine in people without back pain. N Engl J Med 1994; 331(2):69–73.
5. Wilbourn AJ, Aminoff MJ. AAEM Minimonograph 32: the electrodiagnostic examination in patients with radiculopathies. Muscle Nerve 1998;21:1612–31.
6. Cannon DE, Dillingham TR, Miao H, et al. Musculoskeletal disorders in referrals for suspected lumbosacral radiculopathy. Am J Phys Med Rehabil 2007;86(12): 957–61.
7. Lauder TD, Dillingham TR, Andary M, et al. Effect of history and exam in predicting electrodiagnostic outcome among patients with suspected lumbosacral radiculopathy. Am J Phys Med Rehabil 2000;79:60–8.
8. Lauder TD, Dillingham TR, Andary M, et al. Predicting electrodiagnostic outcome in patients with upper limb symptoms: are the history and physical examination helpful? Arch Phys Med Rehabil 2000;81:436–41.
9. Uysal II, Seker M, Karabulut AK, et al. Brachial plexus variations in human fetuses. Neurosurgery 2003;53:676–84.
10. Pellerin M, Kimball Z, Tubbs RS, et al. The prefixed and postfixed brachial plexus: a review with surgical implications. Surg Radiol Anat 2010;32:251–60.
11. Johnson EO, Vekris M, Demesticha T, et al. Neuroanatomy of the brachial plexus: normal and variant anatomy of its formation. Surg Radiol Anat 2010;32:291–7.
12. Loukas M, Lewis RG Jr, Wartman CT. T2 Contributions to the Brachial Plexus. Neurosurgery 2007;60:S13–8.
13. Grana EA, Kraft GH. Lumbosacral Radiculopathies: distribution of electromyographic findings. Muscle Nerve 1992;15(10):1204.
14. Young A, Getty J, Jackson A, et al. Variations in the pattern of muscle innervation by the L5 and S1 nerve roots. Spine 1983;8(6):616–24.
15. Kim YH, Lee PB, Lee CJ, et al. Dermatome variation in lumbosacral nerve roots in patients with transitional lumbosacral vertebrae. Anesth Analg 2008;106(4):1279–83.
16. Fisher MA. Electrophysiology of radiculopathies. Clin Neurophysiol 2002;113: 317–35.
17. Waylonis GW. Electromyographic findings in chronic cervical radicular symptoms. Arch Phys Med Rehabil 1968;49:407–12.
18. Tonzola RF, Ackil AA, Shahani BT, et al. Usefulness of electrophysiological studies in the diagnosis of lumbosacral root disease. Ann Neurol 1981;9(3):305–8.
19. Haig AJ, Tong HC, Yamakawa KS, et al. The sensitivity and specificity of electrodiagnostic testing for the clinical syndrome of lumbar spinal stenosis. Spine 2005; 30(23):2667–76.
20. Coster S, de Bruijn SF, Tavy DL. Diagnostic Value of history, physical examination, and needle electromyography in diagnosing lumbosacral radiculopathy. J Neurol 2010;257:332–7.
21. Yiannikas C, Shahani BT, Young RR. Short-latency somatosensory-evoked potentials from radial, median, ulnar, and peroneal nerve stimulation in the assessment of cervical spondylosis. Arch Neurol 1986;43:1264–71.
22. Tackman W, Radu EW. Observations of the application of electrophysiological methods in the diagnosis of cervical root compressions. Eur Neurol 1983;22: 397–404.
23. American Association of Electrodiagnostic Medicine. Practice parameter for needle electromyographic evaluation of patients with suspected cervical radiculopathy: summary statement. Muscle Nerve 1999;22(Suppl 8):S209–11.

24. Levin KH. Electrodiagnostic approach to the patient with suspected radiculopathy. Neurol Clin 2002;20(2):397–421.
25. Ho YH, Yan SH, Lin YT, et al. Sensory nerve conduction studies of the superficial peroneal nerve in L5 radiculopathy. Acta Neurol Taiwan 2004;13(3):114–9.
26. Richardson JK, Forman GM, Riley B. An electrophysiological exploration of the double crush hypothesis. Muscle Nerve 1999;22:71–7.
27. Stevens JC, Sun S, Beard CM, et al. Carpal tunnel syndrome in Rochester, Minnesota, 1961 to 1980. Neurology 1988;38(1):134–8.
28. Upton ARM, McComas AJ. The double crush in nerve entrapment syndromes. Lancet 1973;2:359–62.
29. Kwon H-K, Hwang M, Yoon D- W. Frequency and severity of carpal tunnel syndrome according to level of cervical radiculopathy: double crush syndrome? Clin Neurophysiol 2006;117:1256–9.
30. Frith RW, Litchy WJ. Electrophysiologic abnormalities of peripheral nerves in patients with cervical radiculopathy. Muscle Nerve 1985;8:613.
31. Morgan G, Wilbourn AJ. Cervical radiculopathy and coexisting distal entrapment neuropathies: double crush syndrome? Neurology 1998;50:78–83.
32. Wilbourn AJ. AAEE Case Report #12: common peroneal mononeuropathy at the fibular head. Muscle Nerve 1986;9:825–36.
33. Radhakrishnan K, Litchy WJ, O'Fallon WM, et al. Epidemiology of cervical radiculopathy. A population-based study from Rochester, Minnesota, 1976 through 1990. Brain 1994;117:325–35.
34. Fisher MA. H reflexes and F waves, fundamentals, normal and abnormal patterns. Neurol Clin 2002;20:339–60.
35. Magladery JW, Porter WE, Park AM, et al. Electrophysiological studies of nerve and reflex activity in normal man. IV. The two-neurone reflex and identification of certain action potentials from spinal roots and cord. Bull Johns Hopkins Hosp 1951;88(6):499–519.
36. Burke D, Gandevia SC, McKeon B. Monosynaptic and oligosynaptic contributions to the human ankle jerk and H-reflex. J Neurophysiol 1984;52(3):435–48.
37. Panizza M, Nilsson J, Hallett M. Optimal stimulus duration for the H reflex. Muscle Nerve 1989;12:576–9.
38. Tsao BE, Levin KH, Bodner RA. Comparison of surgical and electrodiagnostic findings in single root lumbosacral radiculopathies. Muscle Nerve 2003;27:60–4.
39. Kalyon TA, Bilgic F, Ertem O. The diagnostic value of late responses in radiculopathies due to disc herniation. Electromyogr Clin Neurophysiol 1983; 23(3):183–6.
40. Braddom RL, Johnson EW. H reflex: review and classification with suggested clinical uses. Arch Phys Med Rehabil 1974;55(9):412–7.
41. Nishida T, Kompoliti A, Janssen I, et al. H Reflex in S-1 Radiculopathy: latency versus amplitude controversy revisited. Muscle Nerve 1996;19:915–7.
42. Braddom RI, Johnson EW. Standardization of H Reflex and diagnostic use in S1 radiculopathy. Arch Phys Med Rehabil 1974;55:161–6.
43. Desmedt JE, editor. New developments in electromyography and clinical neurophysiology. Basel (Switzerland): Karger; 1973; No. 3. p. 277–93.
44. Nishida T, Levy CE, Lewit EJ, et al. Comparison of three methods for recording tibial H reflex: a clinical note. Am J Phys Med Rehabil 1999;78(5):474–6.
45. Dumitru D. Comparison of three methods for recording tibial H reflex: a clinical note. Am J Phys Med Rehabil 2000;79(3):311–5.
46. Jabre JF. Surface recording of the H-Reflex of the flexor carpi radialis. Muscle Nerve 1981;4:435–8.

47. Christie AD, Inglis JG, Boucher JP, et al. Reliability of the FCR H-Reflex. J Clin Neurophysiol 2005;22(3):204–9.
48. Schimsheimer RJ, Ongerboer de Visser BW, Kemp B. The flexor carpi radialis H-reflex in lesions of the sixth and seventh cervical nerve roots. J Neurol Neurosurg Psychiatr 1985;48:445–9.
49. Eliaspour D, Sanati E, Moqadam MRH, et al. Utility of Flexor Carpi radialis H-reflex in diagnosis of cervical radiculopathy. J Clin Neurophysiol 2009;26(6):458–60.
50. Panayiotoupoulos CP, Chroni E. F-waves in clinical neurophysiology: a review, methodological issues and overall value in peripheral neuropathies. Electroencephalogr Clin Neurophysiol 1996;101:365–74.
51. Toyokura M, Murakami K. F-wave study in patients with lumbosacral radiculopathies. Electromyogr Clin Neurophysiol 1997;37(1):19–26.
52. Scelsa SN, Herskovitz S, Berger AR. The diagnostic utility of F waves in L5/S1 radiculopathy. Muscle Nerve 1995;18(12):1496–7.
53. Tang LM, Schwartz MS, Swash M. Postural effects on F wave parameters in lumbosacral root compression and canal stenosis. Brain 1988;111:207–13.
54. American Association of Electrodiagnostic Medicine. Somatosensory evoked potentials: clinical uses. Muscle Nerve 1999;22(Suppl 8):S111–8.
55. Storm SA, Kraft GH. The clinical use of dermatomal somatosensory evoked potentials in lumbosacral spinal stenosis. Phys Med Rehabil Clin N Am 2004;15:107–15.
56. Kraft GH. Dermatomal somatosensory-evoked potentials in the evaluation of lumbosacral spinal stenosis. Phys Med Rehabil Clin N Am 2003;14:71–5.
57. Snowden ML, Haselkorn JK, Kraft GH, et al. Dermatomal somatosensory evoked potentials in the diagnosis of lumbosacral spinal stenosis: comparison with imaging studies. Muscle Nerve 1992;15:1036–44.
58. Kraft GH. A physiological approach to the evaluation of lumbosacral spinal stenosis. Phys Med Rehabil Clin N Am 1998;9(2):381–9.
59. Hoefer PFA, Guttman SA. Electromyography as a method for determination of level of lesions in the spinal cord. Arch Neurol Psychiatry 1944;51(5):415–22.
60. Tsao B. The electrodiagnosis of cervical and lumbosacral radiculopathy. Neurol Clin 2007;25:473–94.
61. Kraft GH. Fibrillation potential amplitude and muscle atrophy following peripheral nerve injury. Muscle Nerve 1990;13:814–21.
62. Jiang GL, Zhang LY, Shen LY, et al. Fibrillation potential amplitude to quantitatively assess denervation muscle atrophy. Neuromuscul Disord 2000;10:85–91.
63. Dillingham TR, Lauder TD, Andary M, et al. Identifying lumbosacral radiculopathies: an optimal electromyographic screen. Am J Phys Med Rehabil 2000;79:496–503.
64. Lauder TD, Dillingham TR. The cervical radiculopathy screen: optimizing the number of muscles studied. Muscle Nerve 1996;19:662–5.
65. Dillingham TR, Lauder TD, Andary M, et al. Identification of cervical radiculopathies: optimizing the electromyographic screen. Am J Phys Med Rehabil 2001;80:84–91.
66. Lauder TD, Dillingham TR, Huston CW, et al. Lumbosacral radiculopathy screen: optimizing the number of muscles studied. Am J Phys Med Rehabil 1994;73(6):394–402.
67. Buchthal F, Pinell P, Rosenfalck P. Action potential parameters in normal human muscle and their physiological determinants. Acta Physiol Scand 1954;32(2–3):219–29.
68. Crane CR, Krusen EM. Significance of polyphasic potentials in the diagnosis of cervical root involvement. Arch Phys Med Rehabil 1968;49:403–6.

69. LaJoie WJ. Nerve root compression: correlation of electromyographic, myelographic, and surgical findings. Arch Phys Med Rehabil 1972;53:390–2.
70. Dumitru D, Amato AA, Zwarts M, editors. Electrodiagnostic Medicine. 2nd edition. Philadelphia: Hanley & Belfus; 2002. p. 713–76.
71. Dillingham TR, Pezzin LE, Lauder T, et al. Symptom duration and spontaneous activity in lumbosacral radiculopathy. Am J Phys Med Rehabil 2000;79(2): 124–32.
72. Levin KH, Maggiano HJ, Wilbourn AJ. Cervical radiculopathies: comparison of surgical and EMG localization of single-root lesions. Neurology 1996;46(4): 1022–5.
73. Jonsson B, Rundgren A. The peroneus longus and brevis muscles: a roentgenologic and electromyographic study. Electromyography 1971;11(1):93–103.
74. Woods WW, Shea PA. The value of electromyography in neurology and neurosurgery. J Neurosurg 1951;8(6):595–607.
75. Danner R. Occurrence of transient positive sharp wave like activity in the paraspinal muscles following lumbar puncture. Electromyogr Clin Neurophysiol 1982;22: 149–54.
76. Johnson EW, Burkhart JA, Eart WC. Electromyography in postlaminectomy patients. Arch Phys Med Rehabil 1972;53:407–9.
77. Dumitru D, Diaz CA, King JC. Prevalence of denervation in paraspinal and foot intrinsic musculature. Am J Phys Med Rehabil 2001;80:482–90.
78. Fish DE, Shirazi EP, Pham Q. The use of electromyography to predict functional outcome following transforaminal epidural spinal injections for lumbar radiculopathy. J Pain 2008;9(1):64–70.
79. Alrawi MF, Khalil NM, Mitchell P, et al. The value of neurophysiological and imaging studies in predicting outcome in the surgical treatment of cervical radiculopathy. Eur Spine J 2007;16(4):495–500.
80. Tullberg T, Svanborg E, Isaccsson J, et al. A preoperative and postoperative study of the accuracy and value of electrodiagnosis in patients with lumbosacral disc herniation. Spine (Phila Pa 1976) 1993;18(7):837–42.

Mechanical Diagnosis and Therapy for Radiculopathy

Ronald Donelson, MD, MS

KEYWORDS

- Radiculopathy • Mechanical diagnosis and therapy
- Spinal dynamics • Low back pain • McKenzie
- Dynamic disc model

A radiculopathy is a fairly precise diagnosis compared with other painful lumbar disorders. Most low back pain is lumped into the "nonspecific" category for which no definitive diagnosis is possible. However, despite its classic clinical presentation, and even when confirmed by compatible imaging findings of a herniated disc, the radiculopathy diagnosis provides only limited assistance for making decisions about treatment. Surgery, on average, provides quite favorable and predictable relief of radicular pain in a relatively short period of time, while good long-term outcomes with nonsurgical treatment are, again on average, also achievable, with far less risk, but recovery takes much longer.

The phrase "on average" is a key point here. Most data on which clinicians depend for guidance helps with the "average" patient; but individual patients are rarely "average." So how do clinicians and their patients make decisions regarding treatment?

Given varying preferences among patients regarding surgical versus nonsurgical care, shared decision-making programs are widely advocated for assistance,[1] but are still in limited use. These programs focus on presenting a balanced view of the treatment options, with each patient's personal life situation playing an important role in their preference. But do they provide all the information patients would like and therefore should receive?

Nowhere is the high variation in this decision-making more vivid than in the 2003 Medicare data that revealed an eightfold variation in the rates of lumbar laminectomy and discectomy across geographic regions.[2] With no evidence of any variation between these regions regarding the severity of the disc pathology, the ability to make the diagnosis, and patient preferences and satisfaction, the cause of this variation has been attributed to "supply-driven care," specifically a greater supply of surgeons in high-rate areas.

In an effort to address this uncertainty in care, this article describes the management paradigm known as Mechanical Diagnosis and Therapy (MDT)[3] and its

SelfCare First, LLC, 13 Gibson Road, Hanover, NH 03755, USA
E-mail address: donelson@selfcarefirst.com

Phys Med Rehabil Clin N Am 22 (2011) 75–89
doi:10.1016/j.pmr.2010.11.001
1047-9651/11/$ – see front matter © 2011 Elsevier Inc. All rights reserved.

usefulness in decision-making for patients with lumbar radiculopathies, and reviews the relevant literature.

The MDT examination provides information about the characteristics of the pain generator unavailable from any other form of assessment, including more conventional clinical examination tests and even our most advanced forms of spinal imaging. Determining the dynamic mechanical characteristics of a symptomatic herniated lumbar disc enables a far higher level of precision and certainty in decision-making than merely determining the anatomic diagnosis.

This form of dynamic spinal assessment has relevance to both axial pain and sciatica due to its unique ability to determine the potential "reversibility" of symptoms and the substantial evidence that it is related to pain-generating disc pathologies. Such reversibility is very often detected even late in the game, after other forms of conservative treatments have failed. For many, MDT's value is best documented in studies showing that patients who do not receive this form of assessment and treatment often undergo unnecessary surgery.

OVERVIEW OF MECHANICAL DIAGNOSIS AND THERAPY

MDT, the focus of this article, was developed by Robin McKenzie, a New Zealand physiotherapist, 50 years ago. It is well described in many other publications, most notably in McKenzie's textbook.[3]

In essence, this low back management paradigm begins with a unique clinical assessment process that provides precise patient-specific information that directs treatment, which can then be customized to each individual's underlying pain generator. In such individualized care, the "average" patient becomes irrelevant. Abundant evidence makes the case that the clinical findings from this assessment provide much more precise information about the underlying pathology than can be ascertained via conventional clinical testing and our most sophisticated imaging studies.

During the assessment, the patient's history often reveals that their symptoms worsen with one direction of lumbar bending or positioning and improves with another. For example, many individuals' symptoms worsen with lumbar flexion activities such as bending, lifting, sneezing, and prolonged slouched sitting, and improve when erect, most notably while walking.

In addition to the conventional physical examination including neural evaluation, patients' low backs are then essentially taken for a mechanical test-drive by the MDT examiner to determine precisely what aggravates and what relieves their symptoms, looking for a correlation with the patient's history.

Specifically, they are directed to perform, to whatever extent their pain will allow, repeated end-range lumbar test movements and static positioning in different directions of lumbar bending to determine what effect these tests have on the location and intensity of their pain, regardless of whether it is axial pain only or pain referred away from the low back, including radicular pain to the foot (**Fig. 1**). A single direction of testing, that is, the patient's "directional preference," is often elicited that will bring a beneficial pain response in the form of either pain centralization (see later discussion) (**Fig. 2**)[3] in the case of referred or radicular pain, or pain abolition in the case of axial pain. Other directions of testing typically aggravate the pain or even cause it to move further distally, called "peripheralization."

So for those in whom a directional preference is found, the most common preferred direction is lumbar extension, with a smaller number needing laterally directed movements, and a very small group rapidly recovering with lumbar flexion end-range movements.

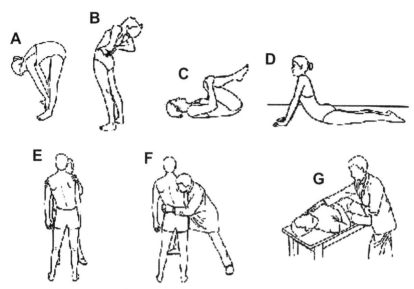

Fig. 1. MDT examination. The standardized physical portion of the MDT assessment has patients perform repeated end-range lumbar movements in both the standing and recumbent positions in lumbar flexion, extension, side-gliding, and rotation. Based on patients' feedback regarding how their pain intensity and location respond to each movement, a directional preference can frequently be identified (A–G). (*From* Donelson R. Is your client's back pain 'rapidly reversible?' Improving low back care at its foundation. Prof Case Manag 2008;13:87–96; with permission.)

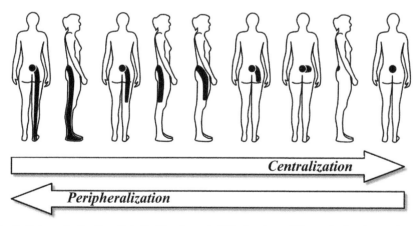

Fig. 2. Pain centralization. Pain that is referred off the lumbar midline, whether just to the paraspinal area or all the way to the foot, can be intentionally centralized back to, or toward, the lumbar midline. This change in pain location is referred to as pain centralization. This pain pattern typically occurs in response to the intentional performance of end-range movements in a single direction. Pain also often peripheralizes, or moves further away from the center of the spine, with movements or positions performed in the opposite direction to lumbar bending. (*From* Donelson R. Is your client's back pain 'rapidly reversible?' Improving low back care at its foundation. Prof Case Manag 2008;13:87–96; with permission.)

Once the patient is evaluated and classified, the MDT examiner then becomes a teacher and coach, helping each patient to learn how to self-manage his or her problem with strategic use of directional exercises every few hours performed in their single beneficial direction (**Fig. 3**). The patients quickly become enabled and empowered to eliminate and then prevent the return of their pain. In addition, they must temporarily avoid bending or positioning the spine for a few days in the opposite direction (see **Fig. 3**).

Patients quickly learn that they are in control of their own pain, by knowing how to turn it on and off, depending on what direction they move or position themselves. This knowledge provides extraordinary insight into the mechanical characteristics of their problem that enables them to either prevent, or at least promptly address, any recurrent pain in the weeks and months ahead, as well as recognize why the pain returned.

TWO INFORMATIVE CLINICAL FINDINGS

Pain centralization and directional preference are 2 clinical findings that are fascinating in large part because they are dynamic. Spine care clinicians are unfamiliar with dynamic mechanisms of pain production and relief. These findings can only be consistently elicited using this MDT dynamic examination.[3] It is also noteworthy that when patients promptly report improvements in their pain intensity and location, they also demonstrate a simultaneous improvement in their lumbar range of motion.

Both centralization and directional preference have been studied extensively for the past 20 years. These studies show that it is highly likely that the spinal loading tests that elicit centralization and directional preference do so because they mechanically influence and alter the underlying pain-generating pathology.

Pain centralization is defined as a progressive retreat of referred or radicular pain back toward or to the center or midline of the lumbar spine, usually as a result of the patient performing repeated end-range movement in a single direction (see

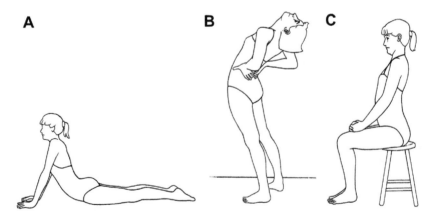

Fig. 3. Extension directional preference. The most prevalent lumbar directional preference is extension, with those same individuals being vulnerable to flexion spinal loading. Repeated press-ups (A) and standing backbends (B) performed to end-range every 2 hours are beneficial extension exercises for this large subgroup, while maintaining a lumbar lordosis while sitting (C) is important between exercise sessions. ((A, B) *From* Donelson R. Is your client's back pain 'rapidly reversible?' Improving low back care at its foundation. Prof Case Manag 2008;13:87–96; with permission; (C) *courtesy of* Ronald Donelson, MD.)

Fig. 2). Other directions of repeated-movement end-range testing in the same patient will not affect the pain or, much more commonly, will aggravate it in some way, such as by increasing its intensity or pushing it further away from the lumbar midline, that is, peripheralization. The single direction of testing that centralizes or often even abolishes the pain is referred to as the patient's directional preference.

RESEARCH

Studies of these two clinical findings are numerous and fall into 3 major categories: prevalence, reliability, and validity. The validity studies are of different types as well: outcome prediction, outcome efficacy, and construct validity. These studies include a wide range of lumbar patients including acute-to-chronic, axial pain only, and sciatica/radiculopathy, and come from at least 7 countries. Some studies focus specifically on radiculopathies.

Prevalence Studies

Since 1990, at least 10 studies have reported on the high prevalence of centralization and directional preference in a wide range of study populations.[4–15] Overall, the reported prevalence of these two findings has been 70% to 87% across acute low back pain studies[16] and 32% to 52% with chronic or radicular patients.[17–21]

Reliability

The value of any clinical test is fundamentally based on its interexaminer reliability. Without reliability there can be no validity, that is, the test is irrelevant. Such studies regarding centralization, directional preference, and MDT patient classification report very acceptable levels of reliability with kappa values greater than 0.6 for identifying centralization and directional preference.[20,22,23] This reliability is superior to any other form of clinical examination, including palpation and observation.[24]

Predictive Validity

Many cohort studies have investigated the impact of identifying centralization and directional preference on patient outcomes. An excellent treatment outcome routinely is reported by patients in whom a directional preference and pain centralization are found, as long as treatment is guided by the patient's directional preference findings.[4,16,22,25–28] In these same studies, outcomes were far less successful in those in whom a directional preference was not found.

But do centralization and directional preference merely identify those who have a good prognosis with most any form of treatment? There are 2 important considerations.

First, if that were the case, there should be no chronic low back pain patients with a directional preference because they would have all recovered with other forms of treatment, or with no particular treatment, long before they became chronic. But the prevalence data show that up to 50% of chronic patients still have a directional preference that, once identified, directs a specific directional exercise treatment defined by the assessment findings that leads to excellent outcomes.[17–21] These patients needed a specific form of directional end-range treatment to correct a problem that had been reversible all along, but was never given the required treatment.

Second, determining whether other treatments might also be beneficial for this large subgroup requires efficacy studies that randomize this large group of directional preference patients to different treatments.

Efficacy Validity

There are now 6 randomized clinical trials (RCTs) targeting this large subgroup of patients who demonstrated the clinical findings of pain centralization and directional preference during their baseline evaluation.[12,29–33] These 6 studies compared the standard MDT treatment of teaching directionally matching exercises and posture modifications with alternative treatments such as stabilization exercises, manual therapy, manipulation, joint mobilization, exercising in the opposite direction to the patient's preference, or guideline-based treatment.

All 6 RCTs show that treating directional preference patients with appropriate directional exercises produced significantly better outcomes compared with any of the treatment alternatives.

While none of these RCTs focused exclusively on patients with radiculopathies, 34% of the Long and colleagues[12] study sample had pain below the knee, half of whom also had neural deficits. Across all directional preference subgroups based on age, duration, and pain location, including those with a radiculopathy, all 6 clinical outcome measures were excellent when directional exercise treatment matched patients' baseline directional preference. For example, patients' self-rated improvement with matching directional exercises was 95% at just 2 weeks, far superior to either guideline-based care (42%) or exercising in the opposite direction from patients' directional preference (23%). Even for these directional preference patients, shown to have such a good prognosis in so many other studies, how they are treated makes a substantial difference. This finding was even clearer when 15% of the patients in the 2 nonmatching study groups, all of whom had a directional preference at their baseline evaluation, reported worsening.

A separately published study reported that a cross-over option was offered to those patients in this same RCT who were initially assigned to an unmatched treatment and did not do well.[27] Of the 96 patients who were then crossed over to matching exercises, 84% reported rapid recoveries after just 2 weeks, once again with significant improvement in all 6 outcome measures.

Construct Validity

There is considerable evidence that the pain-generating structure responsible for most pain centralization and directional preference is the intervertebral disc, regardless of the pain being axial or radiating fully down the leg to the foot with neural deficits.

Numerous imaging and cadaveric studies demonstrate directional mechanical characteristics of intervertebral discs and their nuclei. In normal discs, anterior or flexion loads cause the nucleus to migrate away from the load in a posterior direction, and vice versa with extension loading (**Fig. 4**).[34–40] The nucleus must change its location within the disc to enable the disc to change its shape in order for the spine to bend. The nucleus must move out of the way to enable the edges of the adjacent vertebral bodies to approximate as the spine bends.

Multiple cadaveric studies have shown that posterior disc protrusions and extrusions can be created in otherwise normal discs using either repeated or (ie, excessive) flexion loading.[34,35,37] These lesions resemble the posterior disc pathology seen so commonly in patients whose painful episodes commenced after various forms of flexion activities and postures.

One such study, after creating posterior protrusions, reversed the direction of loading or bending by repeatedly loading these discs in extension.[37] Five of the 11 protrusions then fully reduced, with the nuclei returning to their normal central position within the disc. Those reversible discs were reported to have greater disc height than

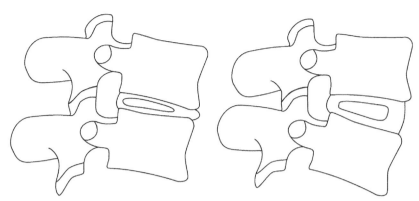

Fig. 4. Dynamic internal disc model. There is considerable evidence that loading a normal lumbar intervertebral disc anteriorly, that is, in flexion, "squeezes" or displaces the nucleus posteriorly. Similarly, when loaded posteriorly, that is, in extension, the nucleus is moved anteriorly. Problems occur when one direction dominates, usually flexion loading, to the extent that excessive displacement occurs that stimulates annular nociception, causes protrusions/herniations, and even leads to compression of an adjacent nerve root. (*Courtesy of* Ronald Donelson, MD.)

those that did not reverse, consistent with the theory that the hydrostatic mechanism within each protruded disc must be sufficiently functional for the nucleus to be reduced or reversed with the extension loading.

Given that both the posterior annulus and lumbar nerve roots are such common sources of back and radiating pain when irritated or compressed respectively by a posterior disc protrusion, it is very plausible that a reduction of the extent of that nuclear displacement, which decompresses those structures using repeated extension loading of the disc, results in both pain centralization of the sciatica and a simultaneous return of the disc's extension range of motion as the obstructing displaced nucleus returns to its normal, more central location within the disc.[3] A posteriorly displaced nucleus obstructs the adjacent vertebral bodies from approximating posteriorly with attempts at extension, until that obstruction is removed by moving it anteriorly using either repeated or sustained extension loading.

End-range repeated movement testing that comprises the MDT assessment seeks to identify the precise direction of bending that reduces the painful nuclear displacement within the symptomatic disc. Often that direction is easy and straightforward to find. Other times it is more complex and requires more than one assessment session to "get it right."[15] Of course, for other patients a directional preference cannot be identified.

Meanwhile, loading a symptomatic disc in the direction opposite to its preference apparently increases the nuclear displacement, causing the pain to either increase or peripheralize.

EVIDENCE THAT IDENTIFYING A DIRECTIONAL PREFERENCE ADDS TO THE PRECISION OF A DISC DIAGNOSIS

Two studies in particular illustrate what the MDT assessment brings to the care of radiculopathy. The first was a retrospective observational study published in 1986 that called attention to the prognostic and therapeutic value of determining whether a patient with lumbar disc prolapse and neurologic deficits exhibited a directional preference, although only the extension direction was tested.[21]

Sixty-seven military personnel with pain radiating to the calf or foot, all with at least one significant physical sign of nerve root irritation (positive straight-leg raising, motor weakness, dermatomal sensory loss, or reflex change), and all with marked reduction in extension range of motion, were hospitalized for surgical consideration because of the severity of their pain and/or failure to respond to outpatient care. All were then tested with end-range extension loading performed in the prone position (see **Fig. 1**) while their symptom response was monitored. Those whose peripheral pain did *not* worsen with this extension testing (n = 35, 52%) were then instructed to perform prone extension exercises frequently (see **Fig. 3**), but only as tolerated, over the next few days. Of these 35, 34 (97%) recovered, 33 within 5 days, and all 35 avoided surgery.

The pain of the remaining 32 (48%) patients peripheralized with their initial extension testing and was unresponsive to any subsequent form of conservative care. All underwent diagnostic imaging and 30 (91%) underwent disc surgery.

Demographic data indicated no difference between these surgical and nonsurgical groups regarding age, symptom location, or neurologic findings. The investigators postulated that this extension treatment was in keeping with a disc nuclear reversal model (just described) as well as the earlier work of Nachemson[41] characterizing the pressure within lumbar discs during extension (normalized to a standing position) as substantially lower than during a relative loss of lumbar lordosis.

Several other points are noteworthy. First and most obvious, a large percentage of patients with compelling clinical evidence of recalcitrant compressive disc disease rapidly reversed their course, even after many other failed treatments. Their effective treatment was determined by their pain response to directional lumbar testing. If not evaluated in this way most, if not all, would have otherwise undergone what this study proved would have been unnecessary disc surgery.

Second, because extension was the only direction tested, there may well have been other patients in this study who also could have avoided surgery and recovered rapidly if they had been evaluated with other directions of end-range testing (eg, lateral-left, lateral-right testing, or rotation) (see **Fig. 1**). These testing directions also elicit the same pain centralization response that enables similar rapid recoveries.[3,7]

Finally, this study illustrates that an anatomic diagnosis of a radiculopathy, normally believed to be precise, was itself completely inadequate for making good treatment decisions. However, by using the dynamic MDT evaluation, substantially more precision was added to the radiculopathy diagnosis by classifying patients into those who can still rapidly reverse and recover with no need for surgery versus those for whom surgery remains an attractive option.

The second study compared the rates of lumbar disc surgery over 10 years in one county in Denmark with those of the rest of Denmark.[42] In the first 5 years the county's rate was lower than the national rate but then was noted to move higher in the sixth year. Many of that county's doctors coincidentally attended a 2-day course on MDT about that time and decided to establish 2 spine clinics in the county to which all patients with low back pain and sciatica would be referred. MDT was a prominent part of the initial evaluation in each clinic. Over the next 4 years, the disc surgery rates in that county dropped by 50%, with initial disc surgeries decreased by two-thirds. The national rates meanwhile remained unchanged. Presumably tens of thousands of Danes in all other counties could have avoided surgery if they too had been given the opportunity to be evaluated for a directional preference.

In both of these studies the need for disc surgery dropped by 50% once patients were provided the opportunity to be evaluated and treated for directional preference. In hindsight, the underlying pathology (disc derangement?) would have been expected to demonstrate a directional preference at the very outset of care when each patient's episode was acute. Further, the centralization prevalence data suggest that the pain generator often loses its ability to reverse over time as the disorder becomes chronic, so there is considerable benefit in assessing these patients as early as possible to reverse and teach those individuals before their underlying disc problem becomes irreversible and requires far more care and associated expense.

So those patients who escaped undergoing surgery could have also avoided most, even all, of their prior care if their directional preference had been identified at the outset of their episode. That prior care typically includes radiographs, advanced imaging, medications, prolonged physical therapy or chiropractic, and diagnostic and therapeutic injections. These interventions are routinely unnecessary in patients found to have a directional preference who are then taught how to predictably and quickly recover.[4,16,22,25–28]

THE PRECISION OF IDENTIFYING A DIRECTIONAL PREFERENCE WITH AXIAL OR REFERRED LOW BACK PAIN OR A RADICULOPATHY

Clinical information and insight gathered from patients found to have a directional preference are not only unique, but add considerable precision to the diagnosis, regardless of whether the anatomic pain source is confirmed or not. What becomes immediately clear to both the examining clinician and the patient is that the underlying pain generator can be changed for the better, even corrected, using simple exercises and posture changes, without having to know the exact tissue source. In other words, the underlying pain source can be improved and corrected without needing to identify it.

The evidence presented earlier that directional preference and pain centralization represent a reduction in painful disc nuclear displacement is compelling, yet it is not a requirement that this disc model be accurate for any single individual to enable recovery.

So, despite anyone's remaining uncertainty about the pain source, very precise information is nevertheless gleaned whenever a directional preference is found. First, the underlying problem is predominately mechanical, not inflammatory. It is also a rapidly reversible or reducible problem, likely caused by something displaced and causing pain. Further, the patient's outcome will be predictably excellent, providing appropriate standardized treatments are used that are also determined during this same assessment.

Regardless of whether the pain is otherwise labeled as radicular or nonspecific, learning a patient has a directional preference provides information that is far more precise and effectual than merely identifying the anatomic source of pain.

NOT EVERYONE HAS A DIRECTIONAL PREFERENCE

Though most do, not every patient has a directional preference. Radiculopathies are typically caused by a herniated disc first stimulating annular nerve endings and then progressing to compress an adjacent nerve root. For reduction of this displacement to occur, the disc's hydrostatic mechanism needs to be sufficiently intact for some patient-specific direction of end-range loading to squeeze the nuclear material back toward the disc's center.[3,43] This process requires the annulus to be intact and competent. However, in cases where the nucleus is extruded, or the annulus is still intact but incompetent, nuclear reduction and pain centralization are no longer achievable and these patients are unable to benefit from MDT treatment, and typically also do not benefit from any other noninvasive form of care.

It is only at this point in care that this small subgroup needs to be imaged to confirm this end-stage disc pathology. Epidural steroids are appropriate, and if there is insufficient improvement surgical excision is indicated. Such surgery can be justified, even recommended, even if the episode is still acute or subacute, due to the benefit of undertaking the surgery before the patient is too physically or psychologically debilitated or before too much work time is lost. Only a precise diagnosis enables making the decision to operate early.

Speedy recoveries, whether nonsurgical or surgical, are in everyone's best interest. The fundamental questions, however, are: who are the patients who can benefit so quickly and definitely from surgery? And who are those who cannot? The MDT assessment can identify these distinctly different subgroups of radiculopathies early, quickly, and reliably.

A 2003 article covered the best evidence at that time for how to manage symptomatic lumbar discs.[43] Considerable detail was provided regarding this dynamic disc model for changing pain location, that is, centralization, directional preference, and patient selection pathways for disc surgery.

FLOW CHART

Fig. 5 portrays the diagnostic pathways that the MDT assessment offers. The large majority of those individuals with either acute or chronic lower back pain have a derangement, that is, something seems to be displaced, causing both pain and obstruction to movement. The great majority is found to have a directional preference

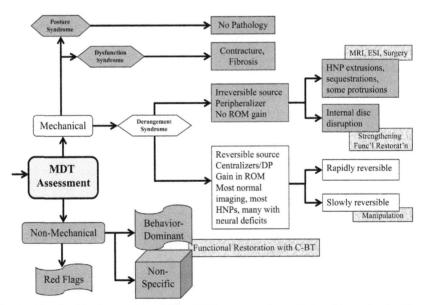

Fig. 5. MDT classification pathways. The MDT assessment can distinguish mechanical from nonmechanical disorders, derangements from nonderangements, and reducible from irreducible derangements. The great majority of patients have reversible derangements (see clear boxes) that rapidly recover if treatment matches their directional preference. C-BT, cognitive-behavioral therapy; DP, directional preference; ESI, epidural steroid injection; HNP, herniated nucleus pulposus; MRI, magnetic resonance imaging; MDT, mechanical diagnosis and therapy; ROM, range of motion. (*Courtesy of* Ronald Donelson, MD.)

that centralizes and abolishes the pain and restores movement. This very large subgroup of patients follows the shaded pathway to a reversible recovery.

The remaining derangements are irreducible. No directional preference or centralization can be found. Many in this group have positive imaging studies for extrusions, sequestrations, and often large protrusions. When a direction of testing cannot be found that centralizes the pain, particularly if every direction of testing seems to increase or peripheralize it, it is safe to conclude that the annulus is completely incompetent, and even if intact, the disc's hydrostatic mechanism is nonfunctional. These are the patients in need of imaging, epidural steroids, and possibly surgery.

Other subgroups can also be identified using the MDT evaluation. The pain of patients with nonmechanical disorders, that is, red flags and dominating psychosocial issues, does not centralize or have a directional preference. It should be noted, however, that many patients with baseline "yellow flags" are in fact centralizers with a directional preference, who recover very well with directional treatments despite their yellow flags.[12,44]

These same MDT assessment methods identify 2 other forms of mechanical back pain. Postural and so-called dysfunction pain are both minor but important syndromes, of much lower prevalence, and thus far poorly documented in the scientific literature as compared with the derangement syndrome. Considerable detail about them can be found in McKenzie's textbook.[3]

RELATIVE ROLES OF MECHANICAL AND INFLAMMATORY FACTORS IN RADICULOPATHY

In unpublished data, 32 Dutch patients with pain below the knee with neural deficits who were making insufficient progress toward recovery, including no directional preference or centralization elicited during an MDT assessment, underwent 3 epidural steroid injections (ESIs).[45] The study design required them to all undergo another MDT assessment after their injections.

Complete relief of pain after the ESIs was reported by 12.5% (n = 4). These subjects were unable to undergo their MDT examination because it requires symptoms that can be monitored.

Forty-seven percent (n = 15) remained noncentralizers with more than half (n = 8) having no pain relief. These patients elected to undergo disc surgery. The remaining noncentralizers (n = 7) had sufficient ESI relief to decide against having surgery.

The remaining 41% (n = 14) were found to now be centralizers with a directional preference. Consequently, their pain was now rapidly reversible using end-range loading that enabled all of them to fully recover. This success increased full recoveries after the ESI from 12.5% with injections alone to 53.5% when postinjection MDT was added.

These latter recoveries clearly required an initial intervention with anti-inflammatory steroids followed by mechanical end-range interventions. Was the inflammatory response to the displaced nucleus and posterior annular disruption/damage that was causing the radiculopathy somehow prohibiting the reduction of the nuclear displacement using end-range loading? Was that same reduction then enabled once the inflammation was addressed to some degree by the ESIs?

Through personal communication, (Hans van Helvoirt, personal communication, 2010) the investigators report their sample size is now more than 70 patients and the distribution of outcomes is similar to their preliminary report.

CLINICIAN AND PATIENT EDUCATION

Articles such as this and continuing medical education courses about MDT have enabled spine clinicians to learn about MDT for the past 20 years. Very few clinicians have been adequately motivated to pursue this education, however. More recently, a book entitled *Rapidly Reversible Low Back Pain* has been well received by a broad range of clinicians who care for patients with low back pain.[46]

Patient education is also critical, so they may know whether they are suffering from acute or chronic, axial or referred low back pain, or radiculopathy. Given the high prevalence of centralization and directional preference, their role in informing and enabling rapid recoveries, and the lack of provision of the MDT assessment to the majority of patients with low back pain and radiculopathy, many more recoveries would no doubt occur if patients were informed of their potential to do so using MDT. A patient information book, *Solving the Mystery: The Key to Rapid Recoveries for Back and Neck Pain*, has been published with just this intent[47] as well as a classic "how-to" self-care book by McKenzie entitled *Treat Your Own Back*.[48]

Shared-decision-making (SDM) educational materials are designed to present a balanced view of patients' treatment options.[1] But how many patients now choose surgery because the outlook with further conservative care, as portrayed in current SDM content, is simply not all that attractive? Current SDM content incorrectly assumes that all available nonoperative care has been used and has failed. But what would patients' preference be if informed of a type of clinical evaluation that, despite prior unsuccessful treatments, could still identify ways that up to 50% with chronic pain could eliminate their own symptoms in a short period of time? Among the majority who had not previously been provided the opportunity to engage MDT, who would not prefer to at least try that pathway before reconsidering surgery, especially when the answer regarding directional preference is so quickly determined? While some would still end up choosing surgery if MDT or a combination of MDT and ESIs failed to help, many would be able to avoid the option of what would otherwise be unnecessary surgery.

SUMMARY

Whether axial lumbar pain, referred pain, or radiculopathy, the clinical findings of pain centralization and directional preference provide precise and highly relevant information about the characteristics of the underlying pain source. These findings are uniquely elicited during a dynamic mechanical test-drive of the lumbar spine using repeated end-range spinal loading tests, that is, the MDT form of patient evaluation as described by McKenzie. Such findings are present in the great majority of patients with acute low back pain and in as many as 50% of patients with chronic low back pain or sciatica.

When found, centralization and directional preference predict that the underlying pain source is reversible. Recovery usually takes place rapidly, using end-range directional exercises and posture modifications that match the directional preference identified during the assessment. Most patients can therefore be quickly empowered to eliminate and then also prevent the return of their own pain.

These clinical findings have been extensively studied in interexaminer reliability studies, outcome predictive and efficacy studies, and anatomic studies of the intervertebral discs. The evidence is substantially supportive in each of these research domains.

Up to 50% of patients with radiculopathies proven to be recalcitrant to other forms of treatment still have reversible disc pathology, meaning their pain can still be centralized and abolished with a single direction of loading of their painful disc. If never provided the opportunity to be adequately tested for these two findings, unnecessary spinal injections and disc surgeries are often undertaken.

Establishing that these painful disc pathologies are rapidly reversible, as well as the means of reversing them, is not possible using our conventional clinical examination or our most advanced imaging. Magnetic resonance imaging (MRI) has considerable difficulty even establishing the anatomic diagnosis of herniated nucleus pulposus independent of the presence of sciatica and neural deficits. Moreover, any MRI diagnosis of a herniated nucleus pulposus is still too imprecise to determine and predict the most effective treatment.

REFERENCES

1. Weinstein J. The missing piece: embracing shared decision making to reform health care. Spine 2000;25(1):1–4.
2. Weinstein J, Lurie J, Olson P, et al. United States' trends and regional variations in lumbar spine surgery: 1992–2003. Spine 2006;31:2707–14.
3. McKenzie R, May S. Mechanical diagnosis and therapy. 2nd edition. Waikanae (New Zealand): Spinal Publications New Zealand Ltd; 2003.
4. Delitto A, Cibulka M, Erhard R, et al. Evidence for an extension-mobilization category in acute low back syndrome: a prescriptive validation pilot study. Phys Ther 1993;73(4):216–28.
5. Donelson R, Aprill C, Medcalf R, et al. A prospective study of centralization of lumbar and referred pain: a predictor of symptomatic discs and annular competence. Spine 1997;22(10):1115–22.
6. Donelson R, Grant W, Kamps C, et al. Pain response to repeated end-range sagittal spinal motion: a prospective, randomized, multi-centered trial. Spine 1991;16(6S):206–12.
7. Donelson R, Grant W, Kamps C, et al, editors. Pain response to end-range spinal motion in the frontal plane: a multi-centered, prospective trial. In: Annual Meeting of International Society for the Study of the Lumbar Spine. Heidelberg (Germany), 1991.
8. Donelson R, Silva G, Murphy K. The centralization phenomenon: its usefulness in evaluating and treating referred pain. Spine 1990;15(3):211–3.
9. Karas R, McIntosh G, Hall H, et al. The relationship between non-organic signs and centralization of symptoms in the prediction of return to work for patients with low back pain. Phys Ther 1997;77(4):354–60.
10. Laslett M, Öberg B, Aprill C, et al. Centralization as a predictor of provocation discography results in chronic low back pain, and the influence of disability and distress on diagnostic power. Spine J 2005;5:370–80.
11. Long A. The centralization phenomenon: its usefulness as a predictor of outcome in conservative treatment of chronic low back pain. Spine 1995;20(23):2513–21.
12. Long A, Donelson R, Fung T. Does it matter which exercise? A randomized controlled trial of exercise for low back pain. Spine 2004;29(23):2593–602.
13. Skytte L, May S, Petersen P. Centralization—its prognostic value in patients with referred symptoms and sciatica. Spine 2005;30:E293–9.
14. Sufka A, Hauger B, Trenary M, et al. Centralization of low back pain and perceived functional outcome. J Orthop Sports Phys Ther 1998;27(3):205–12.
15. Werneke M, Hart DL, Cook D. A descriptive study of the centralization phenomenon. A prospective analysis. Spine 1999;24(7):676–83.
16. Clare H. Missing evidence. Br Med J 2007;332:1430–4.
17. Bogduk N, Lord S. Commentary re: a prospective study of centralization of lumbar and referred pain: a predictor of symptomatic discs and annular competency. Pain Med JI Club JI 1997;3:246–8.

18. Hyodo H, Sato T, Sasaki H, et al. Discogenic pain in acute nonspecific low-back pain. Eur Spine J 2005;14(6):573–7. Available at: http://www.html/fulltext.html. Accessed November 12, 2010.
19. Bronfort G, Haas M, Evans R, et al. Efficacy of spinal manipulation and mobilization for low back pain and neck pain: a systematic review and best evidence synthesis. Spine J 2004;4:335–56.
20. Donelson R. Evidence-based low back care? Br Med J 2007;332(7555):1430–4.
21. Kopp J, Alexander A, Turocy R, et al. The use of lumbar extension in the evaluation and treatment of patients with acute herniated nucleus pulposus, a preliminary report. Clin Orthop Relat Res 1986;202:211–8.
22. Aina S, May S, Clare H. The centralization phenomenon of spinal symptoms— a systematic review. Man Ther 2004;9:134–43.
23. Donelson R. Letter to the editor. J Orthop Sports Phys Ther 2000;30(12):770–3.
24. May S, Littlewood C, Bishop A. Reliability of procedures used in the physical examination of non-specific low back pain: a systematic review. Aust J Physiother 2006;52:91–102.
25. Gotzsche PC. Why we need a broad perspective on meta-analysis: it may be crucially important for patients. BMJ 2000;321:585–6.
26. Donelson R. The reliability of centralized pain response [letter to the editor]. Arch Phys Med Rehabil 2000;81:999–1000.
27. Long A, May S, Fung T. Specific directional exercises for patients with low back pain: a case series. Physiother Can 2008;60:307–17.
28. Chorti A, Chortis A, Strimpakos N, et al. The prognostic value of symptom responses in the conservative management of spinal pain: a systematic review. Spine 2009;34:2686–99.
29. Brennan G, Fritz J, Hunter S, et al. Identifying subgroups of patients with acute/subacute "nonspecific" low back pain. Results of a randomized clinical trial. Spine 2006;31:623–31.
30. Browder D, Childs J, Cleland J, et al. Effectiveness of an extension-oriented treatment approach in a subgroup of patients with low back pain: a randomized clinical trial. Phys Ther 2007;87(12):1–11.
31. Kilpikoski S, Alen M, Paatelma M, et al. Outcome comparison among working adults with centralizing low back pain: secondary analysis of a randomized controlled trial with 1-year follow-up. Adv Physiother 2009;1:1–8.
32. Schenk R, Jazefczyk C, Kopf A. A randomized trial comparing interventions in patients with lumbar posterior derangement. J Manipulative Physiol Ther 2003; 11(2):95–102.
33. Fritz J, Delitto A, Erhard R. Comparison of classification-based physical therapy with therapy based on clinical practice guidelines for patients with acute low back pain: a randomized clinical trial. Spine 2003;28(13):1363–71.
34. Adams M, Hutton W. Prolapsed intervertebral disc. A hyperflexion injury. Spine 1982;7:184–91.
35. Adams M, Hutton W. Gradual disc prolapse. Spine 1985;10:524–31.
36. Fennell A, Jones A, Hukins D. Migration of the nucleus pulposus within the intervertebral disc during flexion and extension of the spine. Spine 1996;21:2753–7.
37. Scannell J, McGill S. Disc prolapse: evidence of reversal with repeated extension. Spine 2009;34:344–50.
38. Schnebel B, Simmons J, Chowning J, et al. A digitizing technique for the study of movement of intradiscal dye in response to flexion and extension of the lumbar spine. Spine 1988;13(3):309–12.

39. Seroussi R, Krag M, Muller D, et al. Internal deformations of intact and enucleated human lumbar discs subjected to compression, flexion, and extension loads. J Orthop Res 1989;7(1):122–30.
40. Shepherd J. In vitro study of segmental motion in the lumbar spine. J Bone Joint Surg Br 1995;77(S2):161.
41. Nachemson A. Disc pressure measurements. Spine 1981;6:93–7.
42. Rasmussen C, Nielsen G, Hansen V, et al. Rates of lumbar disc surgery before and after implementation of multidisciplinary nonsurgical spine clinics. Spine 2005;30:2469–73.
43. Wetzel F, LaRocca H, Lowery G, et al. The treatment of lumbar spinal pain syndromes diagnosed by discography: lumbar arthrodesis. Spine 1994;19(7): 792–800.
44. Werneke M, Hart DL. Centralization phenomenon as a prognostic factor for chronic low back pain and disability. Spine 2001;26(7):758–65.
45. Schepers M, van Helvoirt H, editors. Identification and management of irreducible derangements. Eleventh International Conference on Mechanical Diagnosis and Therapy. Rio de Janeiro (Brazil), August 29, 2009.
46. Donelson R. Rapidly reversible low back pain: an evidence-based pathway to widespread recoveries and savings. Hanover (NH): SelfCare First, LLC; 2007.
47. Donelson R. Solving the mystery: the key to rapid recoveries from back and neck pain. Hanover (NH): SelfCare First, LLC; 2010.
48. McKenzie R. Treat your own back. Waikanae (New Zealand): Spinal Publications; 1997.

The Role of Core Stabilization in Lumbosacral Radiculopathy

David J. Kennedy, MD*, Maureen Y. Noh, MD

KEYWORDS

• Spine • Rehabilitation • Core exercises • Radiculopathy

The prevalence of lumbosacral radiculopathy has been reported to range from 9.9% to 25%.[1] Lumbosacral radiculopathy may arise from a multitude of insults to the spinal nerve as it exits the lumbar spine. The classic description of radiculopathy is compromise of a spinal nerve with resultant pain, weakness, and/or sensory impairment in the distribution of the affected nerve root. This condition may be from direct trauma or from chemical irritation to the affected nerve root. Regardless of the underlying cause, injuries to the lumbar spine have been shown to adversely affect the core musculature and spinal stability.[2] In theory, prolonged injury and pain lead to pain avoidance patterns, which can result in core muscle atrophy, loss of spine flexibility, and altered biomechanics of the spine. These conditions can significantly delay healing or even predispose to secondary injuries. This article reviews current concepts regarding core stability and rehabilitation in the setting of lumbosacral radiculopathy.

OVERVIEW

Core strengthening is widely used for both injury prevention and rehabilitation of the lumbar spine. The muscular core has been described as a box encasing the lumbar spine with the diaphragm on top, pelvic floor on bottom, abdominals anteriorly, and paraspinal and gluteal muscles postreiorly.[3] Core musculature is required for the spine to move freely throughout its entire range of motion, and it also serves as a functional center of the kinetic chain by connecting the upper and lower extremities. The muscles of the pelvic girdle and shoulder, such as the hip abductors and scapular stabilizers, also contribute to core stability through connections to the spine and must not be overlooked in rehabilitation program design. Panjabi[4] first described a model for spinal stability that consists of 3 components: the bone and ligamentous structures, the

Department of Orthopaedics and Rehabilitation, University of Florida, PO Box 112727, Gainesville, FL 32611, USA
* Corresponding author.
E-mail address: kennedj@ortho.ufl.edu

Phys Med Rehabil Clin N Am 22 (2011) 91–103
doi:10.1016/j.pmr.2010.12.002
1047-9651/11/$ – see front matter © 2011 Elsevier Inc. All rights reserved.

muscles surrounding the spine, and the neural input controlling the spine. The bone and ligamentous structures are thought to offer primarily passive stiffness, whereas the core musculature provides for stability through the full range of motion. Neural input allows for specific muscle activation patterns in both planned and unplanned movements. Low-back pain (LBP) has been shown to cause muscle atrophy and altered neural control of the spine musculature.[5] In theory, these effects lead to altered spine biomechanics and thus progression of the degenerative spine cascade.[6] Strengthening and activation of the core musculature are fundamental in the rehabilitation of spine injuries. Several studies have indicated the importance of a few muscles (transversus abdominis [TA] and the lumbar multifidi)[3,7]; however, as noted earlier, evaluation of the kinetic chain and activation of larger muscles are also important in the restoration of normal function and should be addressed in a comprehensive core stabilization program.

ANATOMIC PRINCIPLES OF SPINAL STABILITY
Ligaments and Osseous Structures

The ligaments and osseous structures combine to provide passive stiffness to the spine. The posterior osseous elements of the spine include the zygapophyseal (facet) joints, pedicles, lamina, and pars interarticularis. These structures have limited flexibility and are known to fail with repetitive loading through excessive lumbar flexion and extension.[8] The portion of the spine that is anterior to the spinal cord is composed of the vertebral bodies, the intervertebral disks, and the anterior and posterior longitudinal ligaments. The intervertebral disk is composed of the annulus fibrosis, which encircles the nucleus pulposus. The end plates form a boundary between the disk and vertebral body. The disk can be injured through both compressive and shearing loads that cause injury initially to the end plates and ultimately to the annulus, thereby permitting disk herniation.

The ligaments of the spine include the supraspinous, interspinous, and intertransverse ligaments posteriorly; the elastic ligamentum flavum; and the anterior and posterior longitudinal ligaments on the anterior and posterior sides of the vertebral body, respectively. The anterior and posterior longitudinal ligaments may offer some protection from disk herniation. The combination of a strong anterior longitudinal ligament and limited lumbar extension makes anterior disk herniations rare. The posterior longitudinal ligament provides some protection from a pure posterior herniation, and most herniations occur in the posterolateral direction where the ligament thins and blends with the annulus fibrosis. As a whole, these ligaments seem to provide minimal inherent stability. In fact, it has been demonstrated that a cadaver with bones and ligaments intact but muscles removed buckles under about 9 kg.[9] The role of these ligaments seems to be to provide some kinesthetic awareness as well as to serve as attachments and continuations of the back musculature and fascial planes.

Local Core Musculature

The major source of spinal stability arises from the activation and endurance of the core musculature, which is composed of several muscle groups. The deepest and smallest local spinal muscles include the multifidus, interspinales, and intertransversarii muscles. These muscles span only 2 or 3 spinal segments, and because of their short moment arm, these muscles are not thought to be involved in gross spinal movement. However, the organization of their fibers suggests stabilization of the spine in resisting unopposed lumbar flexion. In addition, their rich composition of muscle spindles suggests that these muscles act as segmental proprioceptive sensors of the spine.[10]

Along with the multifidi, the TA has received attention in its stabilizing role in back pain. The TA runs in a hooplike fashion around the abdomen and attaches broadly to the thoracolumbar fascia.[2] In healthy individuals, the deep fibers of the multifidi and the TA are the first fibers to activate when a limb is moved in response to visual stimulus, firing independently of limb movement direction to control intervertebral movement.[11] In addition to stabilizing the core in preparation for limb movement, the TA has also been shown to increase the stiffness of the lumbar spine and the sacroiliac joints when activated.[7] The multifidi and TA are found to atrophy in people with LBP, and there is evidence that the TA becomes dysfunctional in the setting of LBP.[2,3] Laasonen[12] studied postoperative patients with unilateral LBP and found that paraspinals were 10% to 30% smaller on the affected side when compared with the unaffected side. In patients with LBP and functional inactivity, biopsy results show selective type 2 atrophy of the multifidi and structural changes in type I fibers.[5,13] Antigravity postural muscles have been shown to atrophy to a greater extent than lower extremity muscles in microgravity simulation models.[14]

These changes in muscle composition in healthy individuals who stopped normal repetitive low-level activity patterns are thought to result in transformation of the muscle toward a more fatigable type of muscle fiber.[14,15] All these studies suggest that these muscles are selectively vulnerable to atrophy and dysfunction in the setting of back pain. However, there is some evidence that with exercise training multifidi atrophy can be reversed.[16,17]

Global Muscles Affecting the Core

Lateral to the multifidi is the erector spinae complex, which in the lumbar spine is composed of the longissimus and iliocostalis muscles. These are predominantly thoracic muscles, which attach directly by broad flat tendinous insertions (known as the erector spinae aponeurosis) to the iliac crests. In addition, the lumbar portions of the longissimus and iliocostalis originate from the lumbar vertebrae and attach on the ilium. These muscles provide lumbar extension and increase in lordosis when acting bilaterally and lateral bending when activated unilaterally. These muscles also act in opposition to spinal rotation. Patients with LBP have been shown to have decreased lumbar extensor endurance when compared with controls and to have abnormal trunk flexor to extensor strength ratios.[18–21] The quadratus lumborum lies deep to the erector spinae and spans the regions from the 12th rib to the ilium, with interwoven portions to the expansive thoracolumbar fascia. It has been proposed to be a lumbar extensor as well as to provide lateral bending, and dysfunction can occur with weakness as well as unilateral shortening. The quadratus lumborum can be targeted in physical therapy for lumbar stabilization and is thought to be a key component in a core stabilization program.[22] Anterior to the quadratus lumborum lies the psoas muscles, which arise from the anterior transverse processes and intervertebral disks of the thoracolumbar spine and insert on the femurs, acting primarily as a hip flexor. The psoas muscles may also increase lumbar lordosis when tight and may increase compressive loads of the lumbar spine when acting on the hip. Along with the TA, other circumferential muscles of the abdominal wall include the internal and external obliques. The rectus abdominis is located anteriorly and generally results in flexion of the lumbar spine and is less targeted in a core stabilization program. The internal obliques have a similar orientation of fibers to the TA, but they have received much less attention in the literature. The external obliques act as a check on the anterior pelvic tilt. Together these obliques act to allow for axial rotation and can be thought of as a stabilizing force to counter unwanted axial rotation as well.

The diaphragm and pelvic floor have also been shown to affect the lumbar spine. McGill and colleagues[23] showed that ventilatory challenges may cause diaphragmatic dysfunction and thus lead to increased compressive loads on the lumbar spine. It has also been demonstrated that patients with sacroiliac joint pain have impaired recruitment in both the diaphragm and pelvic floor.[24]

Discussion of the key core muscles is not complete without special attention paid to the thoracolumbar fascia and its associated musculature. This broad multilayered fascial sheath acts as an anchor for multiple muscles and allows for the distribution of kinetic chain forces from the lower to the upper extremities. Caudally it blends with the fascia of the gluteus maximus; cranially its attachments to the latissimus dorsi emphasize the importance of broadening the scope of the rehabilitation treatment plan to include functionally engaging tasks with the upper and lower extremities. In addition, this fascial sheath is also crucial to recall the role of the hip musculature. The hips transfer forces from the lower extremity to the spine during upright activities. Poor endurance in the hip extensors (gluteus maximus) and abductors (gluteus medius) has been noted in people with LBP.[25,26] There has been a demonstrated association of hip extensor strength and subsequent occurrence of LBP in athletes tested in preparticipation physical examination. Asymmetries in hip extensor strength have also been found in female athletes with LBP.[27–29]

Spinal Flexibility

Correction of spinal inflexibilities in addition to muscular imbalances has been advocated as an important component of rehabilitation of the spine. However, evidence is limited regarding the role of spine flexibility and injuries in the setting of lumbosacral radiculopathy. In addition, review of the literature yields conflicting reports as to the role of spine flexibility and range of motion in the treatment of spine injuries.

Several recent studies have suggested that there is no correlation between spinal flexibility and disability or function. Kuukkanen and Mälkiä[30] suggested that in individuals with less severe back pain, flexibility did not play a role in the individuals' overall functional ability. Similarly, a study by Sullivan and colleagues[31] suggested that active lumbar spine flexion should not be used as a treatment goal. Kujala and colleagues[32] looked at a 3-year longitudinal study in which specifically targeted training showed no increase in maximal lumbar extension in adolescent athletes. Moreover, the investigators suggested that aggressive attempts to increase lumbar flexibility could cause unnecessary stress to structures such as the intervertebral disks or the pars interarticularis.

In contrast, other studies have suggested that specific programs can help improve spinal flexibility. Magnusson and colleagues[33] studied a group of patients with chronic LBP and suggested that increased trunk motion could be achieved by participation in a 2-week full-time rehabilitation program. The investigators noted that patients initially demonstrated a pain avoidance behavior but were able to achieve the confidence to recover despite their pain.[33] Kibler and Chandler[34] observed a specific conditioning program that effectively increased the lumbar flexibility in 51 tennis players. Kujala and colleagues[32] also looked at lumbar flexibility and associated LBP between male and female athletes and controls. The investigators found that although no differences were observed between male athletes and controls, the female athletes (gymnasts and figure skaters) had increased overall and lower lumbar range of motion. In addition, decreased lumbar range of motion and decreased maximal extension were predictive of increased LBP in women. Despite the conflicting data regarding the effect of spinal flexibility programs on recovery, it seems reasonable to focus on specific areas of deficits.

Common stretching programs include both spine-specific stretching exercises and lower extremity stretching exercises (**Fig. 1**). Avoidance of aggravating positions in the setting of radiculopathy is prudent and should be addressed by the clinician when initiating a core stabilization program. Generally, avoidance of spinal flexion is advised in the setting of disk herniation, and avoidance of excessive lumbar extension is advised if there is compromise of the neural foramen by the posterior elements.

EXERCISES FOR THE CORE

Designing an appropriate treatment plan depends on astute recognition of the cause and severity of the spinal injury and any secondary comorbidities. Spine rehabilitation generally follows a standard rehabilitation protocol (**Table 1**).

Ability to perform functional activities should incorporate the following transitional phases: (1) pain control, (2) correction of flexibility and strength deficits, (3) maintenance of cardiovascular stamina, and (4) reintegration of functional activities. This section highlights several key exercises used in a core stabilization program.

Core strengthening during an acute injury has not been shown to reduce either the duration or intensity of acute LBP.[35] However, core strengthening may decrease the recurrence of LBP when used at acute onset of symptoms.[2] In individuals with acute nonradiculopathic LBP, there is also strong evidence that prolonged bed rest is detrimental to functional recovery.[36]

Before initiating core strengthening, a short aerobic program of fast walking should be implemented to serve as a warm-up. Fast walking is recommended over slow walking as a warm-up because it has been shown to cause less torque on the lower back.[37] Alternatives include use of an elliptical trainer or treadmill, which can provide

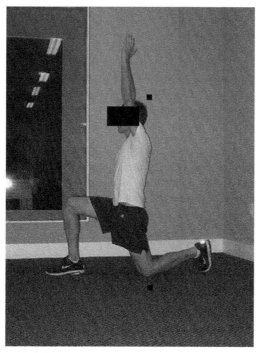

Fig. 1. Left hip flexor stretch.

Table 1
General principles for spinal rehabilitation

Phases	Goals
I. Initial phase: pain control	Antiinflammatory medication Physical modalities Peripheral or axial injections Activity modification
II. Restorative phase: correcting flexibility and strength deficits	Mobilization of soft tissue Stretching exercises to improve trunk and extremity flexibility Strengthening exercises to improve cervical, scapulothoracic, or lumbar stability Maintenance of cardiovascular fitness
III. Integrative phase: functional adaptations	Normalization of spine mechanics Progression toward functional activities
IV. Final phase: maintenance	Pain free Preinjury range of motion and strength

low-impact forms of cardiovascular conditioning. Also, in general, core conditioning is not recommended in the morning because of a theoretical increase of hydrostatic pressure of the disks in the morning.[38] Care should be taken if there is any neurologic weakness due to the radiculopathy, and exercise should not maximally fatigue the affected muscles.

Precise neural control (proprioceptive neuromuscular facilitation) is often disrupted in patients with LBP. As noted earlier, the deep core musculature has been shown in healthy individuals to fire before any limb movement. It has also been demonstrated that these muscles fire significantly later in patients with LBP, often after the prime limb movers such as the deltoid, which suggests inadequate spinal preparation for a planned destabilizing force.[3]

The initial focus of core strengthening should be to facilitate patient awareness of proper motor patterns and reactivation of dormant muscles.

The "cat and camel" and other pelvic translation exercises are effective beginning exercises that allow for spinal segment and pelvic accessory motion before starting more advanced exercises. These exercises may be done in a prone or supine manner as appropriate starting points to train the TA and multifidus, such as performing "abdominal hollowing," which activates the TA. By beginning with these basic movements, the patient can quickly "awaken" the dormant muscles. Biofeedback and verbal cueing may also be used to facilitate neuromuscular activation. These exercises are in nonfunctional positions, and training should quickly transition to functional positions and activities once the proper muscle activation has occurred; however, these can generally be done in a nonpainful range of motion and should assist in exercise compliance.

Exercises can then progress from training isolated muscles to training the core as an integrated unit to facilitate functional activity. The neutral spine has been advocated as a safe place to begin exercise. In addition, lumbar flexion places increased posterior pressure on the intervertebral disk and can exacerbate radicular symptoms, thus a neutral or slightly extension-biased program may be used. Saal and Saal[39] described a dynamic lumbar stabilization program that is among the most widely accepted means of core stabilization. The beginner level exercises incorporate the "big 3" as described by McGill,[21] which includes the curl-up, side bridge (**Fig. 2**), and "bird dog." The bird dog can be advanced from a 4-point stance to a 3-point to

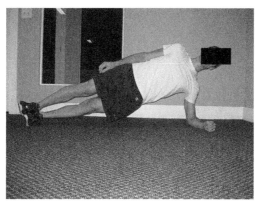

Fig. 2. Side plank exercise.

a 2-point stance. For the higher-level patient, a physioball can be incorporated into the routine (**Fig. 3**). In addition, it is imperative to develop core training in the 3 cardinal planes: sagittal, frontal, and transverse (**Fig. 4**). Research shows that neuromuscular control can be enhanced through combinations of joint stability (cocontraction) exercises, balance training, perturbation (proprioceptive) training, polymeric (jump) exercises, and sports-specific skill training. This can be achieved through a combination of exercises that challenge proprioception via wobble boards, roller boards, and physioballs (**Figs. 5** and **6**).[40]

Deficits in any of these planes of motion can be assessed by physical examination. The multidirectional reach test, the star-excursion balance test (multidirectional excursion assessment in all cardinal planes), and the single leg squat test have all been validated for the assessment of transverse and rotational movements.[41,42] Results from these tests help direct the core training program, focusing on an individual's weaknesses.

Progressive resistance strengthening of the lumbar extensors may be unsafe. The risk of lumbar injury is greatly increased (1) when the spine is fully flexed and (2) when it undergoes excessive repetitive torsion.[43] For example, both the Roman chair and back extensor machines require loads that can be injurious to the lumbar spine.[22] Traditional sit-ups and pelvic tilts also increase compression loads on the lumbar spine and therefore may be unsafe.

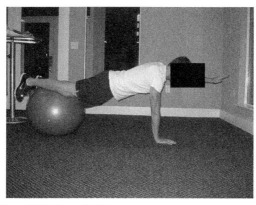

Fig. 3. Triped exercise with balance ball.

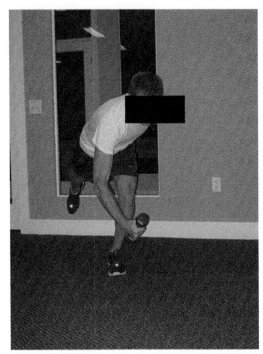

Fig. 4. Triplanar exercise with weights using forward lunge and rotation. (Caution should be taken with advancing to this exercise.)

Reintegration of Functional Activity

The final steps in the rehabilitation process involve integrating the patient into functional activities, taking into account their home, vocational, and avocational needs. Patients and their therapists should develop a home exercise program that builds on the patient's goals and habits to ensure the greatest likelihood of continuation on a maintenance basis. Vocational activities may be simulated, and suggestions for improving biomechanics at work, such as an ergonomic evaluation or evaluation of proper lifting techniques, should be addressed. In addition, patient's avocational activities may include recreational sports, and they should begin these sports-specific motions under the guidance of the trainer or therapist, which allows them to review and correct any biomechanical abnormalities that might impede the recovery process. The progression from basic to more complex motions depends on the subsequent forces placed on the spine.

Efficacy of Exercises

Despite widespread acceptance of a multitude of spine stabilization exercises (ie, Williams flexion exercises), there has been limited study of the utility of these programs in the management of lumbosacral radiculopathy. Various studies have looked at the effect of a treatment exercise program on anatomic changes in spinal muscles. Hides and colleagues[2] assessed the recovery of lumbar multifidi muscles after treatment with an exercise program consisting of isometric contractions of these muscles with cocontraction of the abdominal muscles compared with medical treatment only for individuals after a nonradicular acute lumbar spine injury. The investigators reported

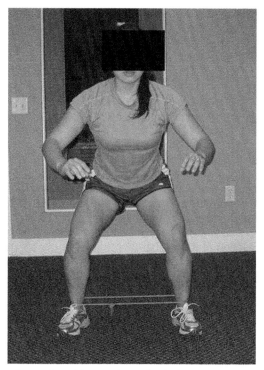

Fig. 5. "Lawn mower" exercise with proprioceptive balance.

improved muscle symmetry and a more rapid and complete recovery of the multifidi muscles in the exercise group. Sung[44] studied the endurance of multifidi muscles and functional status of patients with chronic LBP after participation in a 4-week spinal stabilization program. The investigators noted changes in the multifidi strength in conjunction with other spinal extensor muscles but were unable to attribute the improvement to the multisided muscle alone.

Danneels and colleagues[45] analyzed the effect of 3 different 10-week exercise training programs on the cross-sectional area of the paravertebral muscles in

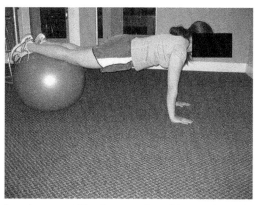

Fig. 6. Medicine ball and core stabilization exercise with proprioceptive balance.

individuals with chronic lumbar spine pain. The investigators suggested that a lumbar stabilization program combined with dynamic resistance training was necessary to restore the size of the paravertebral muscles. These studies suggest that anatomic improvement of the lumbar multifidi muscles could occur through a structured lumbar exercise program.

Other studies have attempted to assess the functional efficacy of a structured strengthening exercise program in individuals with chronic lumbar spine pain. However, there are few prospective, randomized studies. In a prospective study, Käser and colleagues[46] assessed functional improvement in the spine for 3 active exercise treatments (active physical therapy, muscle reconditioning on devices, and low-impact aerobics) over a 3-month period for individuals with chronic lower-back pain. The investigators concluded that significant gains in muscle performance were observed in all 3 exercise groups as noted by a similar increase in isometric strength in all lumbar planar movements, increased activation of the erector spinae during extension testing, and increased endurance testing.[46] Similarly, O'Sullivan and colleagues[47] compared a treatment group using strengthening of the deep abdominal muscles with coactivation of the lumbar multifidi with a control group in individuals with chronic LBP and spondylolisthesis. At 30 months, the treatment group showed a significant improvement in pain, function, range of motion, and abdominal muscle recruitment.[47]

There is a paucity of scientific data with respect to core strengthening as a means to prevent injury. Nadler and colleagues[27] prospectively studied the incidence of LBP in college athletes over 2 seasons. The athletes had a certified strength and conditioning coach implement a core conditioning program into their training regimens before the second season. The male athletes showed a trend but no statistical improvements in LBP occurrence with the implementation of core conditioning. Women showed a non-statistically significant increase in LBP after core training was implemented. This increase in LBP occurred despite measurable increases in hip girdle strength.

These aforementioned studies suggest that a structured strengthening program may be efficacious in the management of spine injuries. Indeed, many of today's spinal rehabilitation programs incorporate control and strengthening of these core muscles of the spine.[48] In the lumbar spine, the program should focus on strength training of the deep intrinsic spinal muscles, such as the lumbar multifidi, with cocontraction of the abdominal muscles. However, more comprehensive, randomized, prospective studies are needed to better assess the efficacy of spinal strengthening exercises in injury treatment and prevention.

SUMMARY

Core stability can be adversely affected in patients with lumbosacral radiculopathy. There is a theoretical basis for core stabilization in injury prevention and treatment. A structured rehabilitation treatment program should focus on correcting inflexibilities and strength deficits as well as improving postural awareness. In addition, integration of the patient's personal goals, including vocational and avocational activities, is paramount in improving compliance with a home exercise maintenance program.

REFERENCES

1. Van Boxem K, Cheng J, Patijn J, et al. 11. Lumbosacral radicular pain. Pain Pract 2010;10(4):339–58.
2. Hides JA, Richardson CA, Jull GA. Multifidus muscle recovery is not automatic after resolution of acute, first-episode low back pain. Spine 1996;21(23):2763–9.

3. Hodges PW. Core stability exercise in chronic low back pain. Orthop Clin North Am 2003;34(2):245–54.
4. Panjabi MM. The stabilizing system of the spine. Part I. Function, dysfunction, adaptation, and enhancement. J Spinal Disord 1992;5(4):383–9 [discussion: 397].
5. Rantanen J, Hurme M, Falck B, et al. The lumbar multifidus muscle five years after surgery for a lumbar intervertebral disc herniation. Spine 1993;18(5):568–74.
6. Krabak B, Kennedy DJ. Functional rehabilitation of lumbar spine injuries in the athlete. Sports Med Arthrosc 2008;16(1):47–54.
7. Richardson CA, Snijders CJ, Hides JA, et al. The relation between the transversus abdominis muscles, sacroiliac joint mechanics, and low back pain. Spine 2002; 27(4):399–405.
8. Standaert CJ, Herring SA. Expert opinion and controversies in sports and musculoskeletal medicine: the diagnosis and treatment of spondylolysis in adolescent athletes. Arch Phys Med Rehabil 2007;88(4):537–40.
9. Crisco JJ, Panjabi MM. The intersegmental and multisegmental muscles of the lumbar spine. A biomechanical model comparing lateral stabilizing potential. Spine 1991;16(7):793–9.
10. Bogduk N, Twomey LT. Clinical anatomy of the lumbar spine. Edinburgh: Churchill Livingstone; 1987.
11. Moseley GL, Hodges PW, Gandevia SC. Deep and superficial fibers of the lumbar multifidus muscle are differentially active during voluntary arm movements. Spine 2002;27(2):E29–36.
12. Laasonen EM. Atrophy of sacrospinal muscle groups in patients with chronic, diffusely radiating lumbar back pain. Neuroradiology 1984;26(1):9–13.
13. Zhao WP, Kawaguchi Y, Matsui H, et al. Histochemistry and morphology of the multifidus muscle in lumbar disc herniation: comparative study between diseased and normal sides. Spine 2000;25(17):2191–9.
14. Deschenes MR, Wilson MH, Kraemer WJ. Neuromuscular adaptations to spaceflight are specific to postural muscles. Muscle Nerve 2005;31(4):468–74.
15. Mannion AF. Fibre type characteristics and function of the human paraspinal muscles: normal values and changes in association with low back pain. J Electromyogr Kinesiol 1999;9(6):363–77.
16. Koumantakis GA, Watson PJ, Oldham JA. Trunk muscle stabilization training plus general exercise versus general exercise only: randomized controlled trial of patients with recurrent low back pain. Phys Ther 2005;85(3):209–25.
17. Koumantakis GA, Watson PJ, Oldham JA. Supplementation of general endurance exercise with stabilisation training versus general exercise only. Physiological and functional outcomes of a randomised controlled trial of patients with recurrent low back pain. Clin Biomech (Bristol, Avon) 2005;20(5):474–82.
18. Jørgensen K, Nicolaisen T. Trunk extensor endurance: determination and relation to low-back trouble. Ergonomics 1987;30(2):259–67.
19. Ebenbichler GR, Oddsson LI, Kollmitzer J, et al. Sensory-motor control of the lower back: implications for rehabilitation. Med Sci Sports Exerc 2001;33(11): 1889–98.
20. Sjölie AN, Ljunggren AE. The significance of high lumbar mobility and low lumbar strength for current and future low back pain in adolescents. Spine 2001;26(23): 2629–36.
21. McGill SM. Low back stability: from formal description to issues for performance and rehabilitation. Exerc Sport Sci Rev 2001;29(1):26–31.
22. McGill SM. Low back exercises: evidence for improving exercise regimens. Phys Ther 1998;78(7):754–65.

23. McGill SM, Sharratt MT, Seguin JP. Loads on spinal tissues during simultaneous lifting and ventilatory challenge. Ergonomics 1995;38(9):1772–92.

24. O'Sullivan PB, Beales DJ, Beetham JA, et al. Altered motor control strategies in subjects with sacroiliac joint pain during the active straight-leg-raise test. Spine 2002;27(1):E1–8.

25. Beckman SM, Buchanan TS. Ankle inversion injury and hypermobility: effect on hip and ankle muscle electromyography onset latency. Arch Phys Med Rehabil 1995;76(12):1138–43.

26. Devita P, Hunter PB, Skelly WA. Effects of a functional knee brace on the biomechanics of running. Med Sci Sports Exerc 1992;24(7):797–806.

27. Nadler SF, Malanga GA, Feinberg JH, et al. Relationship between hip muscle imbalance and occurrence of low back pain in collegiate athletes: a prospective study. Am J Phys Med Rehabil 2001;80(8):572–7.

28. Nadler SF, Malanga GA, DePrince M, et al. The relationship between lower extremity injury, low back pain, and hip muscle strength in male and female collegiate athletes. Clin J Sport Med 2000;10(2):89–97.

29. Nadler SF, Wu KD, Galski T, et al. Low back pain in college athletes. A prospective study correlating lower extremity overuse or acquired ligamentous laxity with low back pain. Spine 1998;23(7):828–33.

30. Kuukkanen T, Mälkiä E. Effects of a three-month therapeutic exercise programme on flexibility in subjects with low back pain. Physiother Res Int 2000; 5(1):46–61.

31. Sullivan MS, Shoaf LD, Riddle DL. The relationship of lumbar flexion to disability in patients with low back pain. Phys Ther 2000;80(3):240–50.

32. Kujala UM, Taimela S, Oksanen A, et al. Lumbar mobility and low back pain during adolescence. A longitudinal three-year follow-up study in athletes and controls. Am J Sports Med 1997;25(3):363–8.

33. Magnusson ML, Bishop JB, Hasselquist L, et al. Range of motion and motion patterns in patients with low back pain before and after rehabilitation. Spine 1998;23(23):2631–9.

34. Kibler WB, Chandler TJ. Range of motion in junior tennis players participating in an injury risk modification program. J Sci Med Sport 2003;6(1):51–62.

35. Hayden JA, van Tulder MW, Malmivaara A, et al. Exercise therapy for treatment of non-specific low back pain. Cochrane Database Syst Rev 2005;3:CD000335.

36. Deyo RA, Diehl AK, Rosenthal M. How many days of bed rest for acute low back pain? A randomized clinical trial. N Engl J Med 1986;315(17):1064–70.

37. Callaghan JP, Patla AE, McGill SM. Low back three-dimensional joint forces, kinematics, and kinetics during walking. Clin Biomech (Bristol, Avon) 1999;14(3): 203–16.

38. Adams MA, Dolan P, Hutton WC. Diurnal variations in the stresses on the lumbar spine. Spine 1987;12(2):130–7.

39. Saal JA, Saal JS. Nonoperative treatment of herniated lumbar intervertebral disc with radiculopathy. An outcome study. Spine 1989;14(4):431–7.

40. Caraffa A, Cerulli G, Projetti M, et al. Prevention of anterior cruciate ligament injuries in soccer. A prospective controlled study of proprioceptive training. Knee Surg Sports Traumatol Arthrosc 1996;4(1):19–21.

41. Kinzey SJ, Armstrong CW. The reliability of the star-excursion test in assessing dynamic balance. J Orthop Sports Phys Ther 1998;27(5):356–60.

42. Olmsted LC, Carcia CR, Hertel J, et al. Efficacy of the star excursion balance tests in detecting reach deficits in subjects with chronic ankle instability. J Athl Train 2002;37(4):501–6.

43. Farfan HF, Cossette JW, Robertson GH, et al. The effects of torsion on the lumbar intervertebral joints: the role of torsion in the production of disc degeneration. J Bone Joint Surg Am 1970;52(3):468–97.
44. Sung PS. Multifidi muscles median frequency before and after spinal stabilization exercises. Arch Phys Med Rehabil 2003;84(9):1313–8.
45. Danneels LA, Cools AM, Vanderstraeten GG, et al. The effects of three different training modalities on the cross-sectional area of the paravertebral muscles. Scand J Med Sci Sports 2001;11(6):335–41.
46. Käser L, Mannion AF, Rhyner A, et al. Active therapy for chronic low back pain: part 2. Effects on paraspinal muscle cross-sectional area, fiber type size, and distribution. Spine 2001;26(8):909–19.
47. O'Sullivan PB, Phyty GD, Twomey LT, et al. Evaluation of specific stabilizing exercise in the treatment of chronic low back pain with radiologic diagnosis of spondylolysis or spondylolisthesis. Spine 1997;22(24):2959–67.
48. Kennedy DJ, Visco CJ, Press J. Current concepts for shoulder training in the overhead athlete. Curr Sports Med Rep 2009;8(3):154–60.

Spinal Manipulation or Mobilization for Radiculopathy: A Systematic Review

Brent Leininger, DC[a],*, Gert Bronfort, PhD, DC[a],
Roni Evans, MS, DC[a], Todd Reiter, MD, DC[b]

KEYWORDS

- Spinal manipulation • Mobilization
- Musculoskeletal manipulations • Radiculopathy
- Peripheral nervous system diseases

This article focuses on spinal manipulative therapy (SMT) and mobilization (MOB) as primary procedures often incorporated with physical therapy and physiotherapeutic modalities in the treatment of radicular signs and symptoms. In North America, SMT/MOB is performed by chiropractors, osteopaths, and physical therapists, with chiropractors accounting for more than 90% of all claims submitted for SMT.[1]

For the purposes of this review, SMT/MOB is defined as an external force applied to the patients by the hand, an instrumental device, or a piece of furniture (eg, table or plinth), resulting in movement and/or separation of the joint articular surfaces with high or low velocity of joint movement.[2,3]

Spine-related arm or leg pain is defined as the constellation of symptoms characterized by unilateral or bilateral radiating pain originating in the cervical or lumbar region and traveling into the extremity with or without neurologic signs.[4,5] For the purpose of this article, spine-related extremity pain includes radiculopathy (loss of sensation, myotomal strength, or muscle stretch reflex), radicular pain (pain in the normal distribution of a spine nerve), and nonradicular radiating pain (pain radiating from the spine into the extremity in a nondermatomal pattern).[6] The pathophysiologic basis for spine-related extremity symptoms is based on 3 proposed mechanisms, (1) biomechanical compression,[7] (2) biochemical/inflammatory mechanism,[8–14] and (3) neovascularization.[15–17]

The authors have nothing to disclose.
[a] Wolfe-Harris Center for Clinical Studies, Northwestern Health Sciences University, 2501 West 84th Street, Bloomington, MN 55431, USA
[b] Inpatient Rehabilitation Center, High Point Regional Health System, 300 Gatewood Avenue, High Point, NC 27262, USA
* Corresponding author.
E-mail address: bleininger@nwhealth.edu

pmr.theclinics.com

EPIDEMIOLOGY

Back-related and neck-related extremity conditions account for greater work loss, recurrences, and costs than uncomplicated low-back and neck pain.[18–21] A review of epidemiologic studies and prevalence estimates of lumbar radiculopathy found the prevalence rates to vary from 1.2% to 43%.[22] Studies that define sciatica as low-back pain (LBP) with leg pain below the knee place the prevalence at 9.9% to 25%.[23–26] Furthermore, the lifetime prevalence of surgery for those with lumbar radiculopathy is 10% compared with 1% to 2% for those with LBP.[27] Cervical spine disorders have been estimated to affect 9% to 12% of the general population.[28] The average annual age-adjusted incidence rates for cervical radiculopathy have been documented as 83.2 per 100,000.[21] Thoracic disk disease and herniation account for less than 2% of all spinal disk surgeries and 0.15% to 4% of all symptomatic spinal disk herniations.[29,30]

PURPOSE

This article presents a comprehensive and up-to-date systematic review of the literature as it relates to the efficacy and effectiveness of SMT or MOB in the management of cervical, thoracic, and lumbar-related extremity pain.

METHODS

This review included randomized controlled trials published before August 10, 2010 in English with no restrictions on methodological quality. A comprehensive search strategy developed by the Cochrane Back Group was used in the following databases: Medline, CINAHL (Cumulative Index to Nursing and Allied Health Literature), Index to Chiropractic Literature, Mantis, and PEDro (Physiotherapy Evidence Database). Studies were included if they listed spine-related extremity symptoms (leg or arm pain, paresthesia, or numbness) as an inclusion criteria, used a spine-related extremity–specific outcome measure (eg, leg or arm pain), or specifically reported results for patients with spine-related extremity symptoms. Studies not specifying spine-related extremity symptoms as inclusion criteria were analyzed separately. Other inclusion criteria for this review included use of SMT and/or MOB of the spine as the primary therapy in at least one intervention group, alone or in combination with other active treatments. Studies in which the effects of manual treatment could be isolated were analyzed separately from those studies in which the effects of the manual treatment could not be isolated. Acceptable comparison groups included no treatment, placebo, and any other type of active intervention. Only patient-reported outcome measures were evaluated. The primary outcome measures for the review were pain, disability, and global perceived effect. Studies not performing between-group analyses for the measured outcomes were not included in the review. Short-term outcomes were defined as occurring within 3 months of the study therapy onset and long-term outcomes were defined as occurring at or after 6 months. The short-term outcome closest to the cessation of treatment was used as the primary short-term outcome for analysis. Actual scores (not change from baseline scores) for the relevant time points were used for analysis when available.

Studies were assessed for quality by 2 reviewers using the risk-of-bias assessment recommended by the Cochrane Collaboration.[31] For a study to be considered low risk of bias, none of the 6 domains recommended by Cochrane (randomization, allocation concealment, blinding, incomplete outcome data, selective outcome reporting, other) may be rated "no" and no more than 2 may be rated "unclear." Because of the inherent complexities involved in blinding manual treatments, trials that did not blind providers or participants were rated unclear, provided that study personnel were unlikely to influence outcome assessments. For a study to be considered moderate risk of bias, a combination of one no and one unclear or 3 unclear ratings were permitted. All studies failing to meet the criteria for low or moderate risk of bias were rated as high risk of bias. The quality of the body of evidence was assessed using the Grading of Recommendations Assessment, Development and Evaluation (GRADE) approach.[31] Using the GRADE approach, high-quality evidence is defined as randomized clinical trials with low risk of bias that provide consistent, direct, and precise results for the outcome. The quality of the evidence was reduced by one level for each of the 6 domains not met (study design, risk of bias, consistency of results, directness, precision, publication bias). If only studies with high risk of bias were present for a given outcome, the quality of evidence was decreased by 2 levels for the risk of bias domain.

All continuous outcomes were analyzed using mean differences after converting to a 0 to 100 scale. Dichotomous outcomes were analyzed for statistical significance using odds ratios. Because of the problems involved with the clinical interpretation of odds ratios, dichotomous outcomes were presented in the tables as absolute risk differences. Statistical pooling was done in the case of 2 or more studies with comparable interventions, study groups, outcomes, and follow-up time points. The pooling methods were either fixed or random effects models, as indicated. Statistical heterogeneity between the studies was assessed using the χ^2 and I^2 statistic (proportion of variation between studies because of heterogeneity). If the null hypothesis of homogeneity was rejected ($P<.1$ or $I^2>40$), the pooled mean difference using a random effects model was calculated. In the case of statistical homogeneity, a fixed effect model was used. When statistical pooling was deemed inappropriate because of clinical heterogeneity, results were reported separately for individual trials. Direction of effect was reported as superior or inferior if the results were statistically significant. Results that failed to reach statistical significance were reported as similar unless the magnitude of effect was greater than 10 points (on a 0–100 scale), which resulted in the direction of effect being reported as favorable or unfavorable.

RESULTS

Our search identified 631 potential studies of which 16 randomized trials with a total of 2132 participants fulfilled the inclusion criteria for the review. A list of excluded trials is provided in **Table 1**. Of these trials, 5 investigated the effectiveness of SMT and/or MOB for cervical spine-related extremity symptoms and 11 investigated that for lumbar-related extremity symptoms. No trials investigating thoracic spine–related extremity symptoms were identified.

Of the included studies, 11 listed spine-related extremity symptoms as inclusion criteria, with 5 of the studies requiring magnetic resonance imaging–confirmed disk herniation or neurologic signs for inclusion.[62–66] Five of the trials included mixed populations of patients with and without spine-related extremity symptoms; 2 of these studies reported separate subgroup analyses,[67,68] and the remaining 3 reported data on spine-related extremity–specific outcomes (eg, leg or arm pain).[69–71] SMT was used in 9 studies, MOB in 5 studies, and a combination of SMT/MOB in 2 studies. Of these studies, 4 focused on patients with acute symptoms, 7 on those with chronic symptoms, and 3 on those with a mix of acute and chronic symptoms. One study did not specify condition duration. Comparison therapies included no treatment, placebo, heat, transcutaneous electrical nerve stimulation, ultrasonography, bed rest, corset, traction, chemonucleolysis, education, and exercise. The specific effect of SMT/MOB could be isolated in 13 of

Table 1
Excluded studies

Excluded Study	Reason
Andersson et al,[32] 1999	Included LBP with or w/o leg symptoms, but no subgroup findings or leg pain–specific outcomes were reported
Arkuszewski,[33] 1986	Quasi-RCT
Blomberg et al,[34,35] 1992/1994	Included LBP with or w/o leg symptoms, but no subgroup findings or leg pain–specific outcomes were reported
Brodin,[36,37] 1983/1982	Included neck pain with or w/o arm symptoms, but no subgroup findings or arm pain–specific outcomes were reported
Bronfort,[38] 1989	Included LBP with or w/o leg symptoms, but no subgroup findings or leg pain–specific outcomes were reported
Bronfort,[39] 1996	Included LBP with or w/o leg symptoms, but no subgroup findings or leg pain–specific outcomes were reported
Bronfort et al,[40] 2000	No between-group analysis performed
Bronfort et al,[41] 2004	No between-group analysis performed
Coppieters et al,[42] 2003	Study included only 1 treatment w/o immediate follow-up
Delitto et al,[43] 1993	Included LBP with or w/o leg symptoms, but no subgroup findings or leg pain–specific outcomes were reported
Dziedzic et al,[44] 2005	Included neck pain with or w/o arm symptoms, but no subgroup findings or arm pain–specific outcomes were reported
Erhard et al,[45] 1994	Included LBP with or w/o leg symptoms, but no subgroup findings or leg pain–specific outcomes were reported
Evans et al,[46] 1978	Included LBP with or w/o leg symptoms, but no subgroup findings or leg pain–specific outcomes were reported
Ferreira et al,[47] 2007	Included LBP with or w/o leg symptoms, but no subgroup findings or leg pain–specific outcomes were reported
Hemmila et al,[48,49] 1997/2002	Included LBP with or w/o leg symptoms, but no subgroup findings or leg pain–specific outcomes were reported
Hoving et al,[50] 2002	Included neck pain with or w/o arm symptoms, but no subgroup findings or arm pain–specific outcomes were reported
Hurwitz et al,[51] 2002	Included neck pain with or w/o arm symptoms, but no subgroup findings or arm pain–specific outcomes were reported
Hurwitz et al,[52] 2002	Included LBP with or w/o leg symptoms, but no subgroup findings or leg pain–specific outcomes were reported
Meade et al,[53] 1990	Excluded participants with suspected radiculopathy
Nwuga,[54] 1982	No patient-reported outcomes; quasi-RCT
Ongley et al,[55] 1987	Included LBP with or w/o leg symptoms, but no subgroup findings or leg pain–specific outcomes were reported
Persson et al,[56] 1997	Manipulation/mobilization was not used on all patients in the treatment group
Seferlis et al,[57] 1998	Included LBP with or w/o leg symptoms, but no subgroup findings or leg pain–specific outcomes were reported
Siehl et al,[58] 1971	No patient-reported outcomes; quasi-RCT
Young et al,[59] 2009	Manipulation/MOB used in both treatment groups
Zaproudina et al,[60] 2009	Included LBP with or w/o leg symptoms, but no subgroup findings or leg pain–specific outcomes were reported
Zylbergold et al,[61] 1981	Inclusion criteria did not specify if participants required leg symptoms

Abbreviations: RCT, randomized controlled trial; w/o, without.

the 16 trials. Overall, the quality of the trials included in the review was poor. Only 1 of the included trials met the criteria for low risk of bias (**Fig. 1**).[65] All but 2 of the trials[70,71] were too dissimilar in terms of patient characteristics, outcome measures, treatments, and comparisons to allow for statistical pooling.

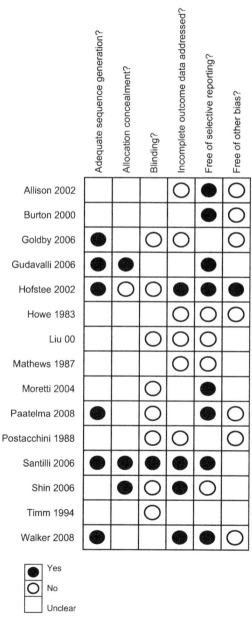

Fig. 1. Risk of bias summary.

Cervical Spine-Related Extremity Symptoms

We identified 5 trials investigating cervical spine–related extremity symptoms that met the inclusion criteria (**Table 2**). All were rated as being at high risk of bias. Three trials isolated the effect of SMT/MOB, whereas 2 trials included combinations of therapies. Howe and colleagues[72] found that a nonsignificant higher proportion of patients receiving SMT plus medication experienced short-term neck, shoulder, and arm pain improvement compared with patients receiving medication alone. Allison and colleagues[62] observed a small, nonsignificant improvement in neck pain and disability in patients receiving MOB and home exercise compared with patients receiving no treatment in the short term. Walker and colleagues[69] found a small nonsignificant improvement in upper extremity pain in patients receiving SMT/MOB plus home exercise compared with usual care plus placebo ultrasonography in the short and long term. Shin and colleagues[63] reported SMT to be superior to traction for neck pain in the short term. Moretti and colleagues[73] observed SMT to be superior to exercise and massage in the short term for pain.

The evidence for SMT and/or MOB for cervical spine–related extremity symptoms is very low in quality for all included comparison therapies. Thus, conclusions regarding effectiveness cannot be made (**Table 3**).

Lumbar Spine–Related Extremity Symptoms

Eleven trials were identified on lumbar spine–related extremity symptoms, which met the inclusion criteria (**Table 4**). Only 1 of the studies[65] was rated as being at low risk of bias and 2 rated as moderate risk[66,67]; the remaining 8 trials were considered to be at high risk of bias. Ten studies isolated the effect of SMT/MOB; one included a combination of SMT and MOB. Santilli and colleagues[65] showed SMT was superior to sham SMT for leg and back pain in the short and long term. Coxhead and colleagues[68] found that SMT was superior to traction, exercise, and corset for pain in the short term. Mathews and colleagues[74,78] observed SMT to be superior to heat for the percentage of improved patients in the short term. Burton and colleagues[64] reported SMT to be superior to chemonucleolysis for back pain and disability in the short term and nonsignificantly better in the long term. Timm[76] found MOB to be superior to passive modalities and no treatment but inferior to exercise for disability in the short term. Goldby and colleagues[70] showed MOB plus general exercise to be inferior to both stabilization exercise and education for leg pain in the short and long term. Paatelma and colleagues[71] found a nonsignificant improvement in leg pain among patients receiving SMT/MOB plus home exercise compared with education in the short and long term. Paatelma and colleagues also found a small, nonsignificant improvement for exercise compared with SMT/MOB plus home exercise for leg pain in the short term, but the groups were similar in the long term.

Gudavalli and colleagues[67] showed that MOB was superior to exercise for pain in the short term. Hofstee and colleagues[66] found that MOB plus exercise and hydrotherapy resulted in similar outcomes for pain and disability compared with education; however, MOB was superior to bed rest for disability in the short term. Liu and Zhang[77] showed SMT to be superior to traction for the percentage of patients improved in the short term. Postacchini and colleagues[75] found SMT to be more favorable than a variety of other treatments; however, statistical significance could not be discerned for all of the comparisons.

Based on the evidence from the 11 trials, there is moderate evidence that SMT is superior to sham SMT for acute leg and back pain in the short and long term. Low-quality or very low–quality evidence for SMT and/or MOB exists for all other

Table 2
Randomized trials of SMT/MOB for cervical spine–related extremity symptoms

Trial (Risk of Bias)	Study Groups (Number of Patients)	Treatments (n)	Results
Howe et al,[72] 1983 (high), acute	G1: SMT-MD + medication (26) G2: medication (26)	1–3	Neck pain improvement (percentage of patients) G1 vs G2: after first treatment, 62[a]; 1 wk, 14; 3 wk, 18 Shoulder pain/paresthesia improvement (percentage of patients) G1 vs G2: after first treatment, 39[a]; 1 wk, 16; 3 wk, 6 Hand pain/paresthesia improvement (percentage of patients) G1 vs G2: after first treatment, 39; 1 wk, 18; 3 wk, 2
Allison et al,[62] 2002[b] (high), chronic	G1: MOB-PT + home exercise (9) G2: no treatment (10)	—	Neck pain G1 vs G2: 2 mo, 4 Neck disability G1 vs G2: 2 mo, 1.4
Walker et al,[69] 2008[c] (high), chronic	G1: SMT/MOB-PT + home exercise (50) G2: usual care + placebo ultrasonography (48)	6 6	Upper extremity pain G1 vs G2: 6 wk, 3; 9 wk, 4.8; 1 y, 3.3
Shin et al,[63] 2006[b] (high), unknown duration	G1: SMT (13) G2: traction (13)	12 12	Neck pain G1 vs G2: 2 wk, 15[a]
Moretti et al,[73] 2004 (high), mixed duration	G1: SMT-PT (40) G2: exercise, massage (40)	2–3 2	Pain G1 vs G2: 2 wk, 38[a]; 6 wk, 54[a]; 3 mo, 58[a]

Results are between-group differences in percentage points unless otherwise specified; positive score indicates advantage for group 1 (G1); underlined outcomes indicate the short-term outcome closest to cessation of treatment.
Abbreviations: G1, group 1; G2, group 2; MD, medical doctor; PT, physiotherapist.
[a] $P \leq .05$ for unadjusted pairwise comparisons.
[b] Studies listed radiculopathy as an inclusion criteria (neurologic signs or magnetic resonance imaging confirmed).
[c] Studies included mixed population of patients with and without arm pain.

Table 3
Evidence of efficacy/effectiveness for cervical spine–related extremity symptoms

SMT and/or MOB	Comparison Intervention	Duration	Outcome	Short Term — Direction of Effect	Short Term — Quality of Evidence[a]	Long Term — Direction of Effect	Long Term — Quality of Evidence[a]
SMT + medication (Howe et al,[72] 1983)	Medication	Acute	Pain (% improved for neck & arm)	Similar	Very low	NA	No evidence
MOB + home exercise (Allison et al,[62] 2002)	No treatment	Chronic	Pain	Similar	Very low	NA	No evidence
SMT + home exercise (Walker et al,[69] 2008)	Usual care + placebo	Chronic	Pain (arm)	Similar	Very low	Similar	Very low
SMT (Shin et al,[63] 2006)	Traction	Unknown	Pain (neck)	Superior	Very low	NA	No evidence
SMT (Moretti et al,[73] 2004)	Exercise + massage	Mixed	Pain	Superior	Very low	NA	No evidence

Superior: significant findings in favor of SMT/MOB group.
Inferior: significant findings in favor of comparison group.
Similar: nonsignificant findings with magnitude below clinical significance.
Favorable: nonsignificant findings in favor of SMT/MOB with magnitude above clinical significance.
Unfavorable: nonsignificant findings in favor of comparison with magnitude above clinical significance.
Abbreviation: NA, not applicable.
[a] GRADE definitions: high, further research is very unlikely to change our confidence in the estimate of effect; moderate, further research is likely to have an important impact on our confidence in the estimate of effect and may change the estimate; low, further research is very likely to have an important impact on our confidence in the estimate of effect and is likely to change the estimate; very low, any estimate of effect is very uncertain.

comparison therapies. Thus, conclusions regarding the effectiveness of SMT/MOB relative to those therapies cannot be made (**Table 5**).

DISCUSSION

There have been several other systematic reviews assessing the effectiveness of SMT/MOB for lumbar spine–related extremity symptoms.[79–85] Overall, the conclusions of our review are consistent with previous reviews. Those reviews published before 2008 found inconclusive or limited evidence for the use of SMT/MOB.[82–85] Of the 3 reviews published after 2008, 2 have concluded that there is moderate evidence for the use of SMT compared with sham.[79,80] One review[81] came to different conclusions, finding the evidence for SMT to be limited; however, it is unclear how the trial by Santilli and colleagues[65] (the only study to be rated as low risk of bias) was taken into account. Differences in review conclusions are likely because of differing methodologies.

Although our review finds moderate evidence for the use of SMT compared with sham SMT for acute lumbar spine–related extremity symptoms, these results should be interpreted cautiously because they are based on the results of only 1 high-quality study.[65] Further, although our review is also in agreement with previous reviews, finding very low–quality or low-quality evidence for SMT/MOB compared with no treatment, passive modalities, education, and exercise for lumbar spine–related extremity symptoms, these findings should also be viewed with caution. Future research, especially if methodologically sound, could easily change the overall estimate of SMT/MOB for lumbar spine–related extremity symptoms.

There are fewer systematic reviews evaluating SMT/MOB for cervical spine–related extremity symptoms.[86–89] Only one of the previous reviews specifically reaches conclusions regarding SMT/MOB for cervical spine–related extremity symptoms. Hurwitz and colleagues[89] found no evidence from any studies that any noninvasive interventions for cervical spine–related extremity symptoms are positively or negatively associated with clinically important outcomes in the short or long term. The current review reaches similar conclusions. We found only very-low evidence for SMT/MOB compared with no treatment, usual care and placebo, traction, and exercise. As a result, the estimate of effect for SMT/MOB in the treatment of cervical spine–related extremity symptoms remains uncertain.

Risks

The decision to use an intervention should also be guided by the potential risk of adverse events or side effects. Most adverse events associated with SMT and MOB are benign in nature and include local discomfort, radiating pain, nausea, dizziness, or tiredness.[90] Estimates of more serious adverse events have remained uncertain because of the limitations of establishing accurate risk estimates for rare events. The most-documented serious adverse event after cervical spine SMT is vertebrobasilar artery (VBA) stroke.[90,91] Estimates of VBA stroke after SMT range from 1 in 200,000 treatments to 1 in several million.[92,93] Recently, Cassidy and colleagues[94] studied the association using a case-control and case-crossover design analyzing more than 100 million person-years of data. The investigators found an increased risk of VBA stroke with SMT in patients younger than 45 years; however, they found a similar increased risk in patients visiting primary care physicians. These findings suggest that increased risk of VBA stroke associated with both provider types is likely due to patients seeking care for headache and neck pain as a result of VBA dissection.

Table 4
Randomized trials of SMT/MOB for lumbar spine–related extremity symptoms

Trial (Risk of Bias)	Study Groups (Number of Patients)	Treatments (n)	Results
Coxhead et al,[68] 1981 (high), chronic	Factorial design, all combinations of 1. SMT-PT, back school, diathermy 2. Traction, back school, diathermy 3. Exercise, back school, diathermy 4. Corset, back school, diathermy	5–10	Pain Main effect of SMT vs no SMT 1 mo, 10[a] Improvement (percentage of patients rating themselves better) Main effect of SMT vs no SMT 1 mo, 9; 4 mo, 5
Mathews et al,[74] 1987 (high), acute	G1: SMT-PT (132) G2: heat (101)	<106	Pain (percentage of patients recovered) G1 vs G2 2 wk, 13[a]
Burton et al,[64] 2000[b] (high), chronic	G1: SMT-DO (20) G2: chemonucleolysis (20)	6–18	Back pain G1 vs G2 2 wk, 12[a]; 6 wk, 12.8[a]; 1 y, 8.6 Leg pain G1 vs G2 2 wk, 0.9; 6 wk, 0.6; 1 y, 2 Disability (RMD) G1 vs G2 2 wk, 15.6[a]; 6 wk, 13.3; 1 y, 5.8
Santilli et al,[65] 2006[b] (low), acute	G1: SMT-DC (53) G2: sham SMT-DC (49)	20 20	Back pain G1 vs G2 1 mo, 8[a]; 6 wk, 18[a]; 3 mo, 18[a]; 6 mo, 16[a] Leg pain G1 vs G2 1 mo, 14[a]; 6 wk, 13; 3 mo, 16[a]; 6 mo, 11[a]

Study	Groups (n)	Sessions	Outcomes
Postacchini et al,[75] 1988[c] (high), mixed duration	G1: SMT-DC (35) G2: mediation (35) G3: massage & diathermy (31) G4: bed rest (14) G5: back school (16) G6: placebo ointment (32)	11–17 10–15 14–21 8 d 4 7–14	Global Improvement Index (pain, disability, finger-floor distance, and straight leg raise) G1 vs G2 3 wk, 7; 6 mo, 6 (acute) 3 wk, 0; 6 mo, 1 (chronic) G1 vs G3 3 wk, 11; 6 mo, 9 (acute) 3 wk, 2; 6 mo, 0 (chronic) G1 vs G4 3 wk, 12; 6 mo, 10 (acute) G1 vs G5 3 wk, 13; 6 mo, 0 (chronic) G1 vs G6 3 wk, 14; 6 mo, 7 (acute) 3 wk, 16; 6 mo, 17 (chronic) (Statistical significance is indeterminate)
Timm,[76] 1996 (high), chronic	G1: MOB-PT (50) G2: heat, TENS, ultrasonography (50) G3: exercise, low technology (50) G4: exercise, high technology (50) G5: no treatment (50)	24 24 24 24	Disability (Oswestry) G1 vs G2 2 mo, 4.9[a] G1 vs G3 2 mo, −17.6[a] G1 vs G4 2 mo, −17[a] G1 vs G5 2 mo, 5[a]
Goldby et al,[70] 2006[c] (high), chronic	G1: MOB-PT, exercise (89) G2: exercise, stabilization (84) G3: education (40)	10 10 1	Leg pain G1 vs G2 3 mo, −8.8[a]; 6 mo, −8.8; 1 y, −6.7 G1 vs G3 3 mo, −11.9[a], 6 mo, −14.6[a], 1 y, −21.2[a] G1 vs G2[d] 3 mo, −7.3[a], 6 mo, −4.6; 1 y, −3 G1 vs G3[d] 3 mo, −4.7; 6 mo, −0.7; 1 y, −5.8

(continued on next page)

Table 4
(continued)

Trial (Risk of Bias)	Study Groups (Number of Patients)	Treatments (n)	Results
Gudavalli et al,[67] 2006[c] (moderate), chronic	G1: MOB-DC (19) G2: exercise (19)	8–16 8–16	Pain G1 vs G2 1 mo, 15.6[a]
Paatelma et al,[71] 2008[c] (high), mixed duration	G1: SMT/MOB-PT, home exercise (45) G2: exercise (52) G3: education (37)	6 6 1	Leg pain G1 vs G2 3 mo, −4; 6 mo, −1; 1 y, 0 G1 vs G3 3 mo, 4; 6 mo, 14; 1 y, 10 G1 vs G2[d] 3 mo, −7.3[a], 6 mo, −4.6; 1 y, −3 G1 vs G3[d] 3 mo, −4.7; 6 mo, −0.7; 1 y, −5.8
Hofstee et al,[66] 2002[b] (moderate), acute	G1: MOB-PT, exercise, hydrotherapy (83) G2: bed rest (84) G3: education (83)	8–16 7 d 1	Leg pain G1 vs G2 1 mo, 2.9; 2 mo, 3.5; 6 mo, 3.2 G1 vs G3 1 mo, 0.6; 2 mo, −0.5; 6 mo, −1.2 Disability (Quebec disability) G1 vs G2 1 mo, 6.9[a], 2 mo, 5.4[a]; 6 mo, 4.5 G1 vs G3 1 mo, 0.9; 2 mo, 1.4; 6 mo, 0.6
Liu & Zhang,[77] 2000 (high), mixed duration	G1: SMT (62) G2: traction (50)	— 28	Pain (percentage of patients improved) G1 vs G2 5 wk, 19.4[a]

Results are between-group differences in percentage points unless otherwise specified. Positive score indicates advantage for group 1 (G1). Underlined outcomes indicate the short-term outcome closest to cessation of treatment.

Abbreviations: DC, chiropractor; DO, osteopath; G1, group 1; G2, group 2; MD, medical doctor; PT, physiotherapist; RMD, Roland Morris Disability Questionnaire; TENS, transcutaneous electrical nerve stimulation.

[a] $P<.05$ for unadjusted pairwise comparisons.

[b] Studies listed radiculopathy as an inclusion criteria (neurologic signs or magnetic resonance imaging confirmed).

[c] Studies included mixed population of patients with and without leg pain.

[d] Pooled estimate from Goldby et al,[70] 2006 and Paatelma et al,[71] 2008.

The potential risks associated with cervical SMT, although rare, are important, and no valid tests exist at present to assess which patients are at risk. Thus, clinicians should take care to responsibly inform patients about the existing uncertainties related to the effectiveness and risk of SMT/MOB for cervical spine–related extremity symptoms. Patients can then make informed choices, consistent with their individual values, as to which noninvasive, and potentially invasive, options to pursue.

Adverse events associated with lumbar spine manipulation are very rare and include disk herniation and cauda equina syndrome.[90] The current risk estimate for lumbar disk herniation after SMT is 1 per million patient visits, and the estimate for cauda equine syndrome is 1 per several million patient visits.[84,95]

Limitations

Conclusions of systematic reviews can vary depending on the methodology chosen to grade the evidence for which there is no absolute standard. We have applied a review methodology consistent with the latest recommendations from authoritative organizations involved in setting standards for systematic reviews.[31] Although a comprehensive search strategy was used, we may not have identified all relevant trials meeting the inclusion criteria. The inclusion of only English language trials is a limitation of the current review; however, the evidence of the potential impact of excluding non-English trials from systematic reviews is conflicting.[96,97] Further, the incidence of randomized trials in non-English journals is declining.[98]

Another limitation of this review is the various definitions of spine-related extremity symptoms that occur in the literature. To avoid disregarding potential evidence, we applied a broad definition, which included radiculopathy, radicular pain, and nonradicular pain originating from the spine. The possibility exists that SMT/MOB has different levels of efficacy/effectiveness for the different categories of extremity pain/symptoms; however, more high-quality trials with specific inclusion criteria are necessary to examine this issue.

The extraction of only follow-up scores instead of changes from baseline is another potential limitation; however, the Cochrane Collaboration recommends primarily using follow-up scores for analysis, if available. The criteria to report the direction of effect for nonsignificant findings are based on arbitrary decisions of clinical importance. However, there is no standard method for determining what constitutes a clinically important group difference in patient-reported outcomes. The decision to report certain magnitudes of effect as clinically important or unimportant has traditionally used effect estimates correlated with individual patient improvement and translated them as being the threshold level for between group importance.[99,100] The current review purposely made no inferences about clinical importance when findings were statistically significant. The decision of clinical importance is complex and depends on many factors, including the benefits, risks, costs of the treatment, and available alternative treatments along with other clinical decision-making criteria.[99]

Clinical Relevance

The findings of the current review have clinical relevance for practitioners treating patients with spine-related extremity symptoms. To enable patients to make informed decisions, clinicians have a responsibility to inform them of the best available research. This includes evidence related to effectiveness, risk, and costs of all available treatment options. It is our opinion that before claims of effectiveness can be made to patients, moderate-quality or high-quality evidence must exist. When only low-quality or very low–quality evidence is present, patients should be informed of the existing uncertainty regarding the effectiveness of the given treatment. Further

Table 5
Evidence of efficacy/effectiveness for lumbar spine–related extremity symptoms

SMT and/or MOB	Comparison Intervention	Duration	Outcome	Short Term		Long Term	
				Direction of Effect	Quality of Evidence[a]	Direction of Effect	Quality of Evidence[a]
SMT[74]	Heat	Acute	Pain (percentage recovered)	Superior	Very low	NA	No evidence
MOB[76]	Heat, TENS, ultrasonography	Chronic	Disability	Superior	Very low	NA	No evidence
SMT/MOB + home exercise[70,71]	Exercise	Chronic & mixed	Pain (leg)	Inferior	Low	Similar	Very low
MOB[67]	Exercise	Chronic	Pain (back)	Superior	Low	NA	No evidence
MOB[76]	Exercise	Chronic	Disability	Inferior	Very low	NA	No evidence
MOB[76]	No treatment	Chronic	Disability	Superior	Very low	NA	No evidence
SMT/MOB + home exercise[70,71]	Education	Chronic & mixed	Pain (leg)	Similar	Very low	Similar	Very low
MOB + exercise[66]	Education	Acute	Pain (leg), disability	Similar	Very low	Similar	Very low
SMT[64]	Chemonucleolysis	Chronic	Pain (leg & back), disability	Superior	Very low	Similar	Very low
SMT[65]	Sham SMT	Acute	Pain (leg & back)	Superior	Moderate	Superior	Moderate
MOB + Exercise[66]	Bed rest	Acute	Pain (leg), disability	Superior	Low	Similar	Very low

	Comparison	Population	Outcome				
SMT[77]	Traction	Mixed	Pain (percentage improved, back)	Superior	Very low	NA	No evidence
SMT[68]	Combination of traction, exercise, corset, diathermy, and education	Chronic	Pain	Superior	Very low	Very low	Similar	Very low
SMT[75]	Medication, massage and diathermy, education, bed rest, placebo gel	Mixed	Global Improvement Index (pain, disability, finger-floor distance, and straight leg raise)	Favorable	Very low	Very low	Similar	Very low

Superior: significant findings in favor of SMT/MOB group.
Inferior: significant findings in favor of comparison group.
Similar: nonsignificant findings with magnitude below clinical significance.
Favorable: nonsignificant findings with magnitude above clinical significance.
Unfavorable: nonsignificant findings in favor of comparison with magnitude above clinical significance.
Abbreviations: NA, not applicable; TENS, transcutaneous electrical nerve stimulation.
[a] GRADE definitions: high, further research is very unlikely to change our confidence in the estimate of effect; moderate, further research is likely to have an important impact on our confidence in the estimate of effect and may change the estimate; low, further research is very likely to have an important impact on our confidence in the estimate of effect and is likely to change the estimate; very low, any estimate of effect is very uncertain.

guidance on how to incorporate research evidence into clinical decision making is provided in a previous report by our group.[101] The goal is to provide the most effective treatments with the least risk and costs that are consistent with patient needs and preferences.

SUMMARY

We found very low–quality evidence for the use of SMT/MOB for cervical spine–related extremity symptoms and no evidence for thoracic spine–related extremity symptoms. The current evidence for other conservative treatments for these conditions is also limited, leaving patients with no clear noninvasive treatment alternatives.[89,102] Consequently, cervical SMT/MOB may be offered as a potential treatment option, once the patient has been informed of the potential risks and benefits of SMT/MOB and other available treatment options.

We found moderate evidence that SMT is more effective than sham SMT for acute lumbar spine–related extremity symptoms. For chronic lumbar spine–related extremity symptoms, the research evidence generally favors SMT/MOB but is of low quality. The current evidence for other conservative treatments for both acute and chronic lumbar spine–related extremity symptoms is generally limited.[79] Consequently, SMT of the lumbar spine is a viable noninvasive treatment option for patients with acute lumbar spine–related extremity symptoms. When risk, cost, and availability of other effective treatment options are considered, SMT/MOB may also be an option for patients with chronic lumbar spine–related extremity symptoms who are amenable to trying a reasonable course of these manual therapies; however, clinicians should remain aware that future high-quality research evidence could easily change what is currently known regarding SMT/MOB effectiveness for lumbar spine–related extremity symptoms.

REFERENCES

1. Shekelle PG. Spinal manipulation. Spine (Phila Pa 1976) 1994;19:858–61.
2. Evans DW, Lucas N. What is 'manipulation'? A reappraisal. Man Ther 2010;15: 286–91.
3. Lee M, Gal J, Herzog W. Biomechanics of manual therapy. In: Dvir Z, editor. Clinical biomechanics. Philadelphia: Churchill Livingstone; 2000. p. 209–38.
4. Spitzer WO. Scientific approach to the assessment and management of activity-related spinal disorders. A monograph for clinicians. Report of the Quebec Task Force on Spinal Disorders. Spine (Phila Pa 1976) 1987;12:S1–59.
5. Atlas SJ, Deyo RA, Patrick DL, et al. The Quebec Task Force classification for spinal disorders and the severity, treatment, and outcomes of sciatica and lumbar spinal stenosis. Spine (Phila Pa 1976) 1996;21:2885–92.
6. Van Akkerveeken PF. Pain patterns and diagnostic blocks. In: Wiesel SW, Weinstein JN, Herkowitz HN, et al, editors. The lumbar spine. 2nd edition. Philadelphia: W.B. Saunders; 1996. p. 105–22.
7. Macnab I. Negative disc exploration. An analysis of the causes of nerve-root involvement in sixty-eight patients. J Bone Joint Surg Am 1971;53:891–903.
8. Johansson A, Hao J, Sjolund B. Local corticosteroid application blocks transmission in normal nociceptive C-fibres. Acta Anaesthesiol Scand 1990;34: 335–8.
9. Ozaktay AC, Cavanaugh JM, Blagoev DC, et al. Phospholipase A2-induced electrophysiologic and histologic changes in rabbit dorsal lumbar spine tissues. Spine (Phila Pa 1976) 1995;20:2659–68.

10. Kang JD, Georgescu HI, McIntyre-Larkin L, et al. Herniated lumbar interverte-bral discs spontaneously produce matrix metalloproteinases, nitric oxide, inter-leukin-6, and prostaglandin E2. Spine (Phila Pa 1976) 1996;21:271–7.

11. Kanemoto M, Hukuda S, Komiya Y, et al. Immunohistochemical study of matrix metalloproteinase-3 and tissue inhibitor of metalloproteinase-1 human interver-tebral discs. Spine (Phila Pa 1976) 1996;21:1–8.

12. Roberts S, Caterson B, Menage J, et al. Matrix metalloproteinases and aggreca-nase: their role in disorders of the human intervertebral disc. Spine (Phila Pa 1976) 2000;25:3005–13.

13. Konttinen YT, Gronblad M, Antti-Poika I, et al. Neuroimmunohistochemical anal-ysis of peridiscal nociceptive neural elements. Spine (Phila Pa 1976) 1990;15: 383–6.

14. Peng B, Wu W, Li Z, et al. Chemical radiculitis. Pain 2007;127:11–6.

15. Furusawa N, Baba H, Miyoshi N, et al. Herniation of cervical intervertebral disc: immunohistochemical examination and measurement of nitric oxide production. Spine (Phila Pa 1976) 2001;26:1110–6.

16. Rudert M, Tillmann B. Detection of lymph and blood vessels in the human inter-vertebral disc by histochemical and immunohistochemical methods. Ann Anat 1993;175:237–42.

17. Peng B, Chen J, Kuang Z, et al. Expression and role of connective tissue growth factor in painful disc fibrosis and degeneration. Spine (Phila Pa 1976) 2009;34: E178–82.

18. Andersson GB. The epidemiology of spinal disorders. In: Frymoyer JW, Ducker TB, Hadler NM, et al, editors. The adult spine: principles and practice. New York (NY): Raven Press; 1997. p. 93–139.

19. Troup JD, Martin JW, Lloyd DC. Back pain in industry. A prospective survey. Spine (Phila Pa 1976) 1981;6:61–9.

20. Valkenburg HA, Haannen HCM. The epidemiology of low back pain. In: White AA III, Gordon SL, editors. American Academy of Orthopaedic Surgeons Symposium on idiopathic low back pain. St Louis (MO): Mosby; 1982. p. 9–22.

21. Radhakrishnan K, Litchy WJ, O'Fallon WM, et al. Epidemiology of cervical rad-iculopathy. A population-based study from Rochester, Minnesota, 1976 through 1990. Brain 1994;117(Pt 2):325–35.

22. Konstantinou K, Dunn KM. Sciatica: review of epidemiological studies and prev-alence estimates. Spine (Phila Pa 1976) 2008;33:2464–72.

23. Svensson HO, Andersson GBJ. Low back pain in 40–47 year old men. I: frequency of occurrence and impact on medical services. Scand J Rehabil Med 1982;14:47–53.

24. Alcouffe J, Manillier P, Brehier M, et al. Analysis by sex of low back pain among workers from small companies in the Paris area: severity and occupational consequences. Occup Environ Med 1999;56:696–701.

25. Miranda H, Viikari-Juntura E, Martikainen R, et al. Physical exercise and muscu-loskeletal pain among forest industry workers. Scand J Med Sci Sports 2001;11: 239–46.

26. Palmer KT, Griffin MJ, Syddall HE, et al. The relative importance of whole body vibration and occupational lifting as risk factors for low-back pain. Occup Environ Med 2003;60:715–21.

27. Frymoyer JW, Pope MH, Clements JH, et al. Risk factors in low-back pain. An epidemiological survey. J Bone Joint Surg Am 1983;65:213–8.

28. Wright A, Mayer TG, Gatchel RJ. Outcomes of disabling cervical spine disorders in compensation injuries. A prospective comparison to tertiary rehabilitation

response for chronic lumbar spinal disorders. Spine (Phila Pa 1976) 1999;24: 178–83.

29. Alvarez O, Roque CT, Pampeti M. Multilevel thoracic disc herniations: CT and MR studies. J Comput Assist Tomogr 1988;12:649–52.

30. Arce CA, Dohrmann GJ. Thoracic disc herniation. Improved diagnosis with computed tomographic scanning and a review of the literature. Surg Neurol 1985;23:356–61.

31. Higgins JPT, Green S, editors. Cochrane handbook for systematic reviews of interventions version 5.0.2. The Cochrane collaboration. Available at: http:// www.cochrane-handbook.org. Accessed September 21, 2010.

32. Andersson GB, Lucente T, Davis AM, et al. A comparison of osteopathic spinal manipulation with standard care for patients with low back pain. N Engl J Med 1999;341:1426–31.

33. Arkuszewski Z. The efficacy of manual treatment in low back pain: a clinical trial. Man Med 1986;2:68–71.

34. Blomberg S, Svardsudd K, Mildenberger F. A controlled, multicentre trial of manual therapy in low-back pain. Initial status, sick-leave and pain score during follow-up. Scand J Prim Health Care 1992;10:170–8.

35. Blomberg S, Svardsudd K, Mildenberger F. A controlled, multicentre trial of manual therapy in low back pain. Initial status, sick leave and pain score during follow-up. J Orthop Med 1994;16:2–8.

36. Brodin H. Cervical pain and mobilization. Acta Belg Med Phys 1983;6:67–72.

37. Brodin H. Cervical pain and mobilization. Manuel Med 1982;20:90–4.

38. Bronfort G. Chiropractic versus general medical treatment of low back pain: a small scale controlled clinical trial. Am J Chiro Med 1989;2:145–50.

39. Bronfort G, Goldsmith CH, Nelson CF, et al. Trunk exercise combined with spinal manipulative or NSAID therapy for chronic low back pain: a randomized, observer-blinded clinical trial. J Manipulative Physiol Ther 1996;19:570–82.

40. Bronfort G, Evans RL, Anderson AV, et al. Nonoperative treatments for sciatica: a pilot study for a randomized clinical trial. J Manipulative Physiol Ther 2000;23:536–44.

41. Bronfort G, Evans R, Maiers M, et al. Spinal manipulation, epidural injections, and self-care for sciatica: a pilot study for a randomized clinical trial. J Manipulative Physiol Ther 2004;27:503–8.

42. Coppieters MW, Stappaerts KH, Wouters LL, et al. The immediate effects of a cervical lateral glide treatment technique in patients with neurogenic cervicobrachial pain. J Orthop Sports Phys Ther 2003;33:369–78.

43. Delitto A, Cibulka MT, Erhard RE, et al. Evidence for use of an extension-mobilization category in acute low back syndrome: a prescriptive validation pilot study. Phys Ther 1993;73:216–22.

44. Dziedzic K, Hill J, Lewis M, et al. Effectiveness of manual therapy or pulsed shortwave diathermy in addition to advice and exercise for neck disorders: a pragmatic randomized controlled trial in physical therapy clinics. Arthritis Rheum 2005;53:214–22.

45. Erhard RE, Delitto A, Cibulka MT. Relative effectiveness of an extension program and a combined program of manipulation and flexion and extension exercises in patients with acute low back syndrome. Phys Ther 1994;74:1093–100.

46. Evans DP, Burke MS, Lloyd KN, et al. Lumbar spinal manipulation on trial. Part I: clinical assessment. Rheumatol Rehabil 1978;17:46–53.

47. Ferreira ML, Ferreira PH, Latimer J, et al. Comparison of general exercise, motor control exercise and spinal manipulative therapy for chronic low back pain: a randomized trial. Pain 2007;131:31–7.

48. Hemmilä HM, Keinanen-Kiukaanniemi SM, Levoska S, et al. Does folk medicine work? A randomized clinical trial on patients with prolonged back pain. Arch Phys Med Rehabil 1997;78:571–7.
49. Hemmilä HM, Keinänen-Kiukaanniemi S, Levoska S, et al. Long-term effectiveness of bone-setting, light exercise therapy, and physiotherapy for prolonged back pain: a randomized controlled trial. J Manipulative Physiol Ther 2002;25:99–104.
50. Hoving JL, Koes BW, de Vet HC, et al. Manual therapy, physical therapy, or continued care by a general practitioner for patients with neck pain. A randomized, controlled trial. Ann Intern Med 2002;136:713–22.
51. Hurwitz EL, Morgenstern H, Harber P, et al. A randomized trial of chiropractic manipulation and mobilization for patients with neck pain: clinical outcomes from the UCLA neck-pain study. Am J Public Health 2002;92:1634–41.
52. Hurwitz EL, Morgenstern H, Harber P, et al. A randomized trial of medical care with and without physical therapy and chiropractic care with and without physical modalities for patients with low back pain: 6-month follow-up outcomes from the UCLA low back pain study. Spine (Phila Pa 1976) 2002;27:2193–204.
53. Meade TW, Dyer S, Browne W, et al. Low back pain of mechanical origin: randomised comparison of chiropractic and hospital outpatient treatment. BMJ 1990;300:1431–7.
54. Nwuga VC. Relative therapeutic efficacy of vertebral manipulation and conventional treatment in back pain management. Am J Phys Med 1982;61:273–8.
55. Ongley MJ, Klein RG, Dorman TA, et al. A new approach to the treatment of chronic low back pain. Lancet 1987;2:143–6.
56. Persson LC, Moritz U, Brandt L, et al. Cervical radiculopathy: pain, muscle weakness and sensory loss in patients with cervical radiculopathy treated with surgery, physiotherapy or cervical collar. A prospective, controlled study. Eur Spine J 1997;6:256–66.
57. Seferlis T, Nemeth G, Carlsson AM, et al. Conservative treatment in patients sick-listed for acute low-back pain: a prospective randomised study with 12 months' follow-up. Eur Spine J 1998;7:461–70.
58. Siehl D, Olson DR, Ross HE, et al. Manipulation of the lumbar spine with the patient under general anesthesia: evaluation by electromyography and clinical-neurologic examination of its use for lumbar nerve root compression syndrome. J Am Osteopath Assoc 1971;70:433–40.
59. Young IA, Michener LA, Cleland JA, et al. Manual therapy, exercise, and traction for patients with cervical radiculopathy: a randomized clinical trial. Phys Ther 2009;89:632–42.
60. Zaproudina N, Hietikko T, Hanninen OO, et al. Effectiveness of traditional bone setting in treating chronic low back pain: a randomised pilot trial. Complement Ther Med 2009;17:23–8.
61. Zylbergold RS, Piper MC. Lumbar disc disease: comparative analysis of physical therapy treatments. Arch Phys Med Rehabil 1981;62:176–9.
62. Allison GT, Nagy BM, Hall T. A randomized clinical trial of manual therapy for cervico-brachial pain syndrome—a pilot study. Man Ther 2002;7:95–102.
63. Shin BC, Kim SD, Lee MS. Comparison between the effects of Chuna manipulation therapy and cervical traction treatment on pain in patients with herniated cervical disc: a randomized clinical pilot trial. Am J Chin Med 2006;34:923–5.
64. Burton AK, Tillotson KM, Cleary J. Single-blind randomised controlled trial of chemonucleolysis and manipulation in the treatment of symptomatic lumbar disc herniation. Eur Spine J 2000;9:202–7.

65. Santilli V, Beghi E, Finucci S. Chiropractic manipulation in the treatment of acute back pain and sciatica with disc protrusion: a randomized double-blind clinical trial of active and simulated spinal manipulations. Spine J 2006;6:131–7.

66. Hofstee DJ, Gijtenbeek JM, Hoogland PH, et al. Westeinde sciatica trial: randomized controlled study of bed rest and physiotherapy for acute sciatica. J Neurosurg 2002;96:45–9.

67. Gudavalli MR, Cambron JA, McGregor M, et al. A randomized clinical trial and subgroup analysis to compare flexion-distraction with active exercise for chronic low back pain. Eur Spine J 2006;15:1070–82.

68. Coxhead CE, Inskip H, Meade TW, et al. Multicentre trial of physiotherapy in the management of sciatic symptoms. Lancet 1981;1:1065–8.

69. Walker MJ, Boyles RE, Young BA, et al. The effectiveness of manual physical therapy and exercise for mechanical neck pain: a randomized clinical trial. Spine (Phila Pa 1976) 2008;33:2371–8.

70. Goldby LJ, Moore AP, Doust J, et al. A randomized controlled trial investigating the efficiency of musculoskeletal physiotherapy on chronic low back disorder. Spine (Phila Pa 1976) 2006;31:1083–93.

71. Paatelma M, Kilpikoski S, Simonen R, et al. Orthopaedic manual therapy, McKenzie method or advice only for low back pain in working adults: a randomized controlled trial with one year follow-up. J Rehabil Med 2008;40:858–63.

72. Howe DH, Newcombe RG, Wade MT. Manipulation of the cervical spine—a pilot study. J R Coll Gen Pract 1983;33:574–9.

73. Moretti B, Vetro A, Garofalo R, et al. Manipulative therapy in the treatment of benign cervicobrachialgia of mechanical origin. Chir Organi Mov 2004;89:81–6.

74. Mathews JA, Mills SB, Jenkins VM, et al. Back pain and sciatica: controlled trials of manipulation, traction, sclerosant and epidural injections. Br J Rheumatol 1987;26:416–23.

75. Postacchini F, Facchini M, Palieri P. Efficacy of various forms of conservative treatment in low back pain. A comparative study. Neuro Orthoped 1988;6: 28–35.

76. Timm KE. A randomized-control study of active and passive treatments for chronic low back pain following L5 laminectomy. J Orthop Sports Phys Ther 1994;20:276–86.

77. Liu J, Zhang S. Treatment of protrusion of lumbar intervertebral disc by pulling and turning manipulations. J Tradit Chin Med 2000;20:195–7.

78. Mathews W, Morkel M, Mathews J. Manipulation and traction for lumbago and sciatica: physiotherapeutic techniques used in two controlled trials. Physiother Pract 1988;4:201–6.

79. Jordan J, Konstantinou K, O'Dowd J. Herniated lumbar disc. Clin Evid (Online) 2009;2009:pii 1118.

80. Hahne AJ, Ford JJ, McMeeken JM. Conservative management of lumbar disc herniation with associated radiculopathy: a systematic review. Spine (Phila Pa 1976) 2010;35:E488–504.

81. Lawrence DJ, Meeker W, Branson R, et al. Chiropractic management of low back pain and low back-related leg complaints: a literature synthesis. J Manipulative Physiol Ther 2008;31:659–74.

82. Luijsterburg PA, Verhagen AP, Ostelo RW, et al. Effectiveness of conservative treatments for the lumbosacral radicular syndrome: a systematic review. Eur Spine J 2007;16:881–99.

83. Chou R, Huffman LH. Nonpharmacologic therapies for acute and chronic low back pain: a review of the evidence for an American Pain Society/American

College of Physicians clinical practice guideline. Ann Intern Med 2007;147: 492–504.

84. Assendelft WJ, Bouter LM, Knipschild PG. Complications of spinal manipulation: a comprehensive review of the literature. J Fam Pract 1996;42:475–80.

85. Bronfort G. Spinal manipulation: current state of research and its indications. Neurol Clin 1999;17:91–111.

86. Gross A, Miller J, D'Sylva J, et al. Manipulation or mobilisation for neck pain. Cochrane Database Syst Rev 2010;1:CD004249.

87. D'Sylva J, Miller J, Gross A, et al. Manual therapy with or without physical medicine modalities for neck pain: a systematic review. Man Ther 2010;15:415–33.

88. Miller J, Gross A, D'Sylva J, et al. Manual therapy and exercise for neck pain: a systematic review. Man Ther 2010;15:334–54.

89. Hurwitz EL, Carragee EJ, van der Velde G, et al. Treatment of neck pain: noninvasive interventions: results of the Bone and Joint Decade 2000–2010 Task Force on Neck Pain and Its Associated Disorders. Spine (Phila Pa 1976) 2008;33:S123–52.

90. Rubinstein SM. Adverse events following chiropractic care for subjects with neck or low-back pain: do the benefits outweigh the risks? J Manipulative Physiol Ther 2008;31:461–4.

91. Ernst E. Adverse effects of spinal manipulation: a systematic review. J R Soc Med 2007;100:330–8.

92. Michaeli A. A reported occurrence and nature of complications following manipulative physiotherapy in South Afrika. Aust J Physiother 1993;39:309–15.

93. Haldeman S, Carey P, Townsend M, et al. Arterial dissections following cervical manipulation: the chiropractic experience. CMAJ 2001;165:905–6.

94. Cassidy JD, Boyle E, Cote P, et al. Risk of vertebrobasilar stroke and chiropractic care: results of a population-based case-control and case-crossover study. Spine (Phila Pa 1976) 2008;33:S176–83.

95. Haldeman S, Rubinstein SM. Cauda equina syndrome in patients undergoing manipulation of the lumbar spine. Spine (Phila Pa 1976) 1992;17:1469–73.

96. Moher D, Pham B, Lawson ML, et al. The inclusion of reports of randomised trials published in languages other than English in systematic reviews. Health Technol Assess 2003;7:1–90.

97. Juni P, Holenstein F, Sterne J, et al. Direction and impact of language bias in meta-analyses of controlled trials: empirical study. Int J Epidemiol 2002;31: 115–23.

98. Galandi D, Schwarzer G, Antes G. The demise of the randomised controlled trial: bibliometric study of the German-language health care literature, 1948 to 2004. BMC Med Res Methodol 2006;6:30.

99. Dworkin RH, Turk DC, McDermott MP, et al. Interpreting the clinical importance of group differences in chronic pain clinical trials: IMMPACT recommendations. Pain 2009;146:238–44.

100. Dworkin RH, Turk DC, Wyrwich KW, et al. Interpreting the clinical importance of treatment outcomes in chronic pain clinical trials: IMMPACT recommendations. J Pain 2008;9:105–21.

101. Bronfort G, Haas M, Evans R, et al. Effectiveness of manual therapies: the UK evidence report. Chiropr Osteopat 2010;18:3.

102. Australian Acute Musculoskeletal Pain Guidelines Group. Evidence-based management of acute musculoskeletal pain. Bowen Hills (Queensland): Australian Academic Press Pty Ltd; 2003.

Pharmaceutical Therapy for Radiculopathy

Christopher J. Visco, MD[a],*, David S. Cheng, MD[a],
David J. Kennedy, MD[b]

KEYWORDS

• Radiculopathy • Pharmaceutical
• Nonsteroidal antiinflammatory drugs • Medications

Radiculopathy often presents clinically with a neuropathic component. The neuronal damage or irritation is felt as radicular pain. In the lumbar spine, this condition may be called sciatica by the lay press when the pain is radiating down the back of the leg. However, the term sciatica is misleading because radiating pain may occur without nerve irritation, and neuronal pain can present in different dermatomes and myotomes.

The pain pathway is a complex feedback loop of peripheral and central pathways, inflammatory mediators, and receptor modulation.[1] Hence, the use of pharmaceuticals in radiculopathy can be multifaceted, targeting any of these potential components of the neuropathic pain response to improve function. A variety of pain medications have been developed to intercept differing areas of the pain pathway, including opioids, nonsteroidal antiinflammatory drugs (NSAIDs), corticosteroids, antidepressants, antiepileptics, muscle relaxants, and topical treatments. The decision to initiate one of these pharmaceutical agents is complementary to the entire treatment plan. Consideration is given to pain severity and chronicity, secondary functional limitations due to pain, and future enrollment in physical therapy or further interventions.

The relatively recent focus on pain as a fifth vital sign has helped hasten the evolution of oral analgesia. Research, development, manufacturing, and marketing of pharmaceuticals for analgesia make up a multibillion dollar industry with physicians near the end of the line helping guide patients to the correct treatment plan. Unfortunately, there are no medications developed specifically for radiculopathy, and there are currently no consensus guidelines to recommend a uniformly accepted treatment

[a] Department of Rehabilitation and Regenerative Medicine, Columbia University College of Physicians and Surgeons, New York, NY 10032, USA
[b] Department of Orthopaedics and Rehabilitation, University of Florida College of Medicine, c/o Marlene Gardner, 4101 NW 89th Boulevard, Gainesville, FL 32606, USA
* Corresponding author.
E-mail address: cv2245@columbia.edu

Phys Med Rehabil Clin N Am 22 (2011) 127–137
doi:10.1016/j.pmr.2010.11.003
1047-9651/11/$ – see front matter © 2011 Elsevier Inc. All rights reserved.

algorithm. The general lack of consensus guidelines may stem from the lack of robust available literature on the topic. Therefore, the decision to initiate a treatment must be tailored to the individual with the choice of analgesic agent based on the patient's comorbid medical conditions and specific pain complaints, including frequency, quality, and severity. Careful identification of the cause along with proper subgrouping of patients may lead to more effective use of medications and resources. For instance, those with chronic back pain have little chance of sustained recovery if a medication is used as initial therapy.[2,3] However, NSAIDs seem to be effective in the acute phase of radiculopathy. Systemic corticosteroids do not seem to be indicated for any group of patients with low-back pain.[4] Muscle relaxants are not indicated as the first-line treatment of low-back pain but can be a good adjunct in the acute phase. Also, alterations in neural pathways occur in those with chronic pain, including central sensitization.[5,6] That development, combined with a peripheral increase in sodium and calcium channels, leads to increased excitability throughout the entire pathway and abnormal transmissions perceived as pain by the patient.[7,8] Therefore, the medication choice may vary depending on the chronicity, severity, and character of pain.

In general, analgesic agents can be divided into 2 major categories. First-line treatments include those medications that are efficacious with favorable safety profiles, low cost, and sometimes over-the-counter access. The second category encompasses medications that are helpful in a specific subgroup of patients but otherwise has questionable efficacy or significant adverse effects. This article reviews the literature for each major category of commonly used medication in the treatment of painful radiculopathy.

NONOPIOID ANALGESIA

Acetaminophen is used extensively for the treatment of low-back pain and may also be used for radiculopathy. The analgesic properties of acetaminophen stem from the inhibition of central prostaglandin synthesis.[9(p150)] Acetaminophen is particularly useful in older persons with multiple comorbidities because opioids can increase fall risk, and selective NSAIDs may increase the risk of cardiovascular disease, bleeding, gastrointestinal (GI) irritation, and renal toxicity.[10,11] Despite the lack of evidence supporting the efficacy of acetaminophen for treating radiculopathy, the American College of Physicians recommends using acetaminophen as a first-line option for low-back pain because of its relatively benign safety profile.[12] Acetaminophen's onset of action is rapid, and it is considered an excellent medication for mild to moderate pain.[2] Because acetaminophen is metabolized by the liver, excessive acetaminophen ingestion is associated with hepatotoxicity. The current recommended dose is less than 4 g/d. If the patient responds to a small dose, one may consider increasing the total daily dose of acetaminophen before adding another medication. Dosages higher than the 650 mg standard do not seem to have incremental benefit, so there may be a ceiling effect.[9(p150)] Caution should be advised against concomitant alcohol consumption to avoid the rare complication of fulminate hepatic necrosis.[13]

OPIOIDS

Opioids remain one of the most versatile and useful medications for analgesia. Opioids are the workhorses of severe pain treatment but they are also polarizing in the social and political realm because of their abuse and addiction potential. The decision to initiate opioid analgesia can be a boon or burden to the patient depending on the management of adverse effects, which can be profound. The potency of analgesia is dose dependent and often limited only by the adverse effects for the patient.[4]

Opioids have been demonstrated to be helpful in neuropathic pain conditions.[14] Eisenberg and colleagues[15] had shown in an 8-week trial that intermediate opioid treatment significantly decreased neuropathic pain compared with gabapentin. In a randomized, double-blind, placebo-controlled study by Gilron and colleagues,[16] the greatest symptomatic improvement was from gabapentin combined with morphine. However, most of these studies were performed in patients with neuropathic pain from causes other than lumbar or cervical radiculopathy.[17,18] In studies of nerve root–related symptoms and neuropathic pain, opioids did not demonstrate significant improvement in symptoms, even when combined with the antineuropathic medications.[5,19,20]

Common adverse effects from opioid medications range from somnolence and mild GI upset to nausea, vomiting, and constipation. Constipation occurs via the same mechanism of analgesia, μ receptor activation.[9(p113)] Some adverse effects can be anticipated and easily managed. For instance, stool softeners should be routinely offered to anyone starting to use opioid analgesia to help mitigate the inevitable constipation associated with these medications. Histamine-releasing effects, such as pruritus, and anticholinergic effects, such as hypotension and bradycardia, can also be seen.[19,21] When severe, patients may experience respiratory suppression and die. Caution should be used in the elderly because opioids can worsen gait disturbances and increase fall risk. Although the risk of addiction is relatively low, physical dependence happens frequently for patients who take these medications chronically, and patients should be counseled accordingly.[22] The long-term effects of chronic opioid use may be associated with the development of tolerance and immunologic and endocrine changes.

Tramadol is a synthetic molecule with 2 moieties, on one side a weak opioid and on the other, a weak serotonin-norepinephrine reuptake inhibitor (SNRI). Therefore, tramadol activates the opioid μ receptor and inhibits the reuptake of norepinephrine and serotonin. The molecule then undergoes hepatic metabolism and renal excretion. Tramadol has demonstrated only minimal efficacy over placebo alone.[2] Common adverse effects include nausea, dizziness, somnolence, and headache. In a study of 7198 patients on tramadol for chronic pain, 7.1% experienced unspecific central nervous system (CNS) irritation and coordination disorders, 5.3% had dizziness, 4.8% had nausea, and another 2.4% complained of sedation.[23] Caution should be taken with patients on a tricyclic antidepressant (TCA) because of an increased risk of seizures. Seizure risk is rare (<1%) but increased with a history of alcohol abuse, stroke, brain injury, or renal dysfunction.[9(p126)] Administering multiple serotonergic medications may lead to serotonin syndrome.[21]

NSAIDs

NSAIDs may be indicated for short-term use to treat inflammation and pain caused by radiculopathy. NSAIDs have both analgesic and antiinflammatory properties. The mechanism of action of NSAIDs is cyclooxygenase (COX) and leukotriene inhibition, preventing the conversion of arachidonic acid to prostaglandins. NSAIDs vary in dosage, potency, and degree of COX-1 and COX-2 inhibition. In addition to mediating pain and inflammation, COX-1 is associated with platelet aggregation, gastric protection, and renal and vascular smooth muscle activity.[9(p144)] Therefore COX-1 inhibition can have adverse effects on those systems. One common demarcation used for NSAIDs is selective (preferentially COX-2) versus nonselective (both COX-1 and COX-2) inhibition. Commonly used nonselective NSAIDs include naproxen, ibuprofen, and diclofenac. Meloxicam, etodolac, and nabumetone are semiselective. Collectively, nonselective NSAIDs are indistinguishable from each other in terms of tolerability but may have some slight differences in efficacy.[24] However, nonselective NSAIDs are not indicated for chronic use, particularly in the elderly because of the risk of GI irritation, ulceration, and bleeding (COX-1 inhibitory effects). Concomitant use of a proton pump inhibitor can decrease the gastric adverse effects. COX-2, or selective NSAIDs, allows for fewer GI effects but may increase cardiotoxicity and should also be avoided in the elderly population. Limited studies have been conducted specifically for the use of COX-2 in radiculopathy; however, meloxicam has been shown to have a significant improvement in sciatic pain at both the 7.5 mg and 15 mg dose when taken for a week compared with placebo. Meloxicam was also shown to be superior in efficacy to diclofenac.[25] Overall, compared with controls, NSAIDs as a class has been shown to improve symptoms of low-back pain, but the literature is less robust for radiculopathy.[20]

Oral Steroids

Although the efficacy of epidural corticosteroid injections in radicular pain has been elucidated,[26,27] the role of oral and intravenous steroids remains unclear. There are various theories as to the mechanism of effect of corticosteroids because they demonstrate effects beyond pure antiinflammation. In the case of spinal stenosis, steroids may help mitigate the inflammation of neural elements and address the chemical radiculitis.[28] In addition to the antiinflammatory mechanism, steroids may also block the development of prostaglandins centrally from the dorsal horn neurons (so-called central sensitization). Steroids may also directly stabilize the membrane of nociceptive C-fibers, blocking transmission and preventing ectopic discharge.[29,30] In a double-blind controlled clinical trial by Holve and Barkan, 27 subjects were assigned to a 9-day tapering course of prednisone versus placebo for acute radiculopathy. Although there seemed to be a trend of improved and faster pain relief, the results did not reach statistical significance.[31] Older studies of intravenous and intramuscular steroid showed that it was no better than placebo. The adverse effects of these medications were also poorly described.[32–34] Nonetheless a short duration (<3 weeks) of low-dose corticosteroid use has relatively few complications regardless of the method of administration.[35] Long-term steroid use, on the other hand, has been linked to hyperglycemia, GI ulceration, weight gain, insomnia, hypertension, hypoadrenocorticism, osteoporosis, friable skin, depression, immunosuppression, osteoporosis, muscular weakness, and rarely avascular necrosis of the femoral head.

Neuromodulatory Medications

Neuromodulatory medications can be largely divided into 2 categories, antidepressants and membrane stabilizers or anticonvulsants. Within the antidepressant category there are selective serotonin reuptake inhibitors (SSRIs), SNRIs, and TCAs.

SSRIs are commonly used as an adjuvant to manage emotional components of neuropathic pain. Despite the fact that SSRIs do not seem to have primary analgesic properties, they seem to have a role in treating pain,[9(p125)] which may be because of the affective component of pain and an extremely high frequency of psychiatric illness in the pain population.[36–38] Psychiatric illness is associated with worse pain intensity and related disability.[39–41] There are data that citalopram and paroxetine may be beneficial in the treatment of peripheral neuropathic pain; however, there is no evidence of their efficacy in radiculopathy.[22] Common adverse effects include GI bleeding and headaches. The risk of GI bleeding is increased with concomitant NSAID use.[19] To mitigate the adverse events, gradually increasing the dose may be helpful. As a class, SSRIs undergo hepatic metabolism and may alter the CYP-450 pathway.[42]

A rare but well-documented drug-drug interaction to consider is serotonin syndrome. This syndrome can arise from the use of multiple serotonergic agents including, SSRI, SNRI, TCA, and tramadol. Clinically, patients may present with profuse sweating, tremor, agitation, hyperthermia, tachycardia, and hypertension. This syndrome is a potentially lethal complication that may lead to cerebral vasoconstriction, stroke, and even death.

SNRIs modulate both serum serotonin as well as norepinephrine levels by inhibiting reuptake. The addition of norepinephrine reuptake inhibition has been shown to improve analgesia and decrease the likelihood of depression remission.[43,44] Duloxetine (Cymbalta) and venlafaxine (Effexor) are the best-studied medications in this group. Duloxetine has been shown to be effective in diabetic peripheral neuropathy according to 3 randomized control trials. However, the use of duloxetine in other types of neuropathy has not been validated.[22] Duloxetine has a relatively favorable safety profile with nausea being the most common symptom. At higher dosages (60 mg twice daily), there is a higher incidence of somnolence, hyperhidrosis, anorexia, vomiting, and constipation.[1] As opposed to duloxetine, which affects serotonin and norepinephrine equally, venlafaxine essentially behaves as an SSRI at low dose and as an SNRI at higher doses. Again, there is literature to suggest that venlafaxine is efficacious in diabetic peripheral neuropathy and other painful polyneuropathies. There are, however, no data to recommend the use of venlafaxine in other central neuropathic pain syndromes.[22] Several adverse effects are seen with venlafaxine, including nausea, withdrawal/discontinuation syndrome, sexual dysfunction, and dose-dependent cardiovascular problems. In fact, in one study, as many as 5% of patients on venlafaxine developed electrocardiographic changes.[22] Thus, one must use discretion in patients with preexisting cardiac conditions.

Discovered in the 1950s, TCAs are so named because they contain 3 rings of atoms. TCAs nonselectively inhibit the reuptake of serotonin and norepinephrine to provide analgesia. TCAs are also theorized to stabilize nerve membranes.[1] TCAs are inexpensive, dosed once daily, and well studied to relieve neuropathic pain, all with similar efficacy. The relatively rapid analgesic effect of TCAs is thought to be separate from the antidepressant properties.[14] However, there is no evidence documenting its utility in chronic low-back pain or radicular pain. Adverse effects, well studied and documented, include sedation, falls, anticholinergic effects (dry mouth, urinary retention, constipation), orthostatic hypotension, cardiac conduction blocks, arrhythmias, and myocardial infarction. For this reason, the use of TCAs has been supplanted by the newer and safer SSRIs and SNRIs. When TCA use is necessary, screening electrocardiograms are routinely recommended for patients older than 40 years before initiating therapy.[22] For those patients in whom a TCA is appropriate, the adverse effect profile can be considered as the deciding factor. For instance, amitriptyline and imipramine tend to be more sedating, and nortriptyline is less anticholinergic.[36]

Antiepileptic medications inhibit voltage-gated sodium and calcium channels to decrease excitatory neurotransmitter (glutamate) release, to potentiate γ-aminobutyric acid (GABA) transmission, and to stabilize neural membranes. Carbamazepine has not been studied extensively, but small studies have found effectiveness for sciatica.[45] Studies of the use of carbamazepine in other peripheral neuropathic conditions have produced variable results.[14] Although gabapentin and pregabalin are structurally related to GABA, they do not bind to $GABA_A$ or $GABA_B$ receptors. Instead, gabapentin and pregabalin are calcium channel blockers with α_2/δ_1 subunits. The most significant distinction between these drugs is that pregabalin has an excellent bioavailability and linear pharmacokinetics. In a study by Yildirim and colleagues,[46] 50 patients with lumbosacral radiculopathy who were randomly assigned to oral gabapentin ranging from 900 to 3600 mg/d or to placebo for 8 weeks were described. Those who received gabapentin were shown to have improved motor and sensory function, lumbar flexion range of motion (P<.001), and pain at rest. Similarly, a prospective study of 1304 subjects with inadequately managed cervical and lumbar radiculopathy were started on either pregabalin as monotherapy or adjuvant therapy versus acetaminophen, NSAIDs, or tramadol. The investigators found a significant reduction of pain severity and resource consumption in those receiving pregabalin.[47] Both gabapentin and pregabalin are fairly well tolerated and have similar adverse effect profiles consisting of dizziness, somnolence, peripheral edema, and vertigo/ataxia.[1]

Topiramate and lamotrigine block sodium channels, which helps to decrease the excitability of actively firing neurons. Topiramate and lamotrigine also block glutamate, the excitatory neurotransmitter responsible for pain transmission.[9(p137)] In addition, topiramate enhances GABA, and in one study, topiramate produced small analgesic effects at 200 mg in those with imaging-confirmed radiculopathy.[48] Another study cited that at 500 mg daily, topiramate reduces pain and improves mood and quality of life.[49] Lamotrigine is commonly used in trigeminal neuralgia; however, it has a high incidence of undesirable adverse effects such as paresthesia, fatigue, weakness, sedation, and diarrhea. In a small study of 14 patients published in the *European Journal of Pain* in 2003, lamotrigine at 400 mg/d improved intractable radicular pain.[50] Levetiracetam is a relatively new antiepileptic whose mechanism of action is still unclear. The use of this antiepileptic was found to improve pain scores, activity, ambulation, and mood in 26 patients with radiological and electrophysiological evidence of lumbar radiculopathy at 1500 mg twice a day (P≤.001). Associated adverse effects include sedation, GI upset, headache, and blurry vision.[51]

Oral Muscle Relaxants

Benzodiazepine medications are commonly thought to work indirectly; relaxing the muscle spasm that is caused by underlying injury by binding to the GABA receptor. These medications are administered under the presumption that the muscle spasm itself is painful. Benzodiazepines are also CNS depressants that act on the limbic system, brainstem reticular formation, and cortex. For this reason they are also useful for anxiety and panic attacks.[52] A Cochrane review found skeletal muscle relaxants better than placebo 2 to 4 days after the acute onset of low-back pain.[2] Other articles specifically studying cyclobenzaprine and tizanidine also support these findings.[2,53,54] However, there is no evidence that this effect translates to radiculopathy. In one study by Asiedu and colleagues,[55] the direct pain-relieving properties of benzodiazepines were explored. Carbonic anhydrase, which normally assists in replenishing intracellular neuronal mediators, was inhibited after intrathecal administration of midazolam with acetazolamide. This administration resulted in decreased neuropathic pain from a peripheral nerve injury. Tizanidine was administered in an escalating dose from 6 to 36 mg total daily for an 8-week period in another noncontrolled study of 23 patients with neuropathic pain, showing improvements in quality of life and pain.[53]

The side effects from muscle relaxants may be their most desirable attribute. The sedative effect is powerful and occurs in up to 50% of subjects in a variety of studies.[53,54,56] Patients with insomnia in the setting of low-back pain can take these medications at night to assist with sleep. Based on available data, there is currently no role for muscle relaxants as a first-line agent in lumbosacral radiculopathy.

Anti–tumor Necrosis Factor α

Early evidence is conflicting regarding the role of anti–tumor necrosis factor α agents in radiculopathy. Most studies are on open-label use and not controlled, which limits the utility of the data. Smaller studies without controls often show improvements in pain and function because of the natural history of most radicular pain. For example one uncontrolled study of 10 subjects with sciatica treated with infliximab revealed improved radicular pain and return to work in all patients.[57] That said, a follow-up study of 40 patients in a placebo-controlled study revealed no difference between groups because both improved.[58] At present, larger, controlled, and randomized studies are lacking in this area.

Topical Treatments

Topical treatments offer an adjunct or alternative to orally administered medications. Palliation of neuropathic pain may also occur with topical use of the medications already discussed. However, topical treatments have been studied primarily in those with pain from postherpetic neuralgia or diabetic peripheral neuropathy. By extrapolation, a more proximal peripheral nerve lesion due to a herniated disk affecting the ventral ramus should respond accordingly, but this is not borne in the literature. In randomized, double-blind, controlled studies, lidocaine 2.5% and 5% gel and patch have been effective in alleviating localized allodynic and nonallodynic pain complaints.[14,21,22] The patch is particularly useful when an occlusive dressing is desirable. Because of the action on sodium channels and possible effects on cardiac conduction, topical lidocaine should be avoided in those on antiarrhythmic medications. Lidocaine undergoes hepatic clearance, and thus its long-term use is not safe in those with severe hepatic dysfunction because blood levels of lidocaine elevate steadily. This observation is in contrast to that with topical diclofenac. This NSAID offers a systemic absorption of less than 10% when applied topically compared with an equivalent oral dose.[21]

Derived from chili peppers, capsaicin cream offers an interesting alternative in peripheral neuropathic pain control. Again, because studies have focused primarily on postherpetic neuralgia and diabetic peripheral neuropathy, the ability to justify the use of capsaicin in neuropathic pain caused by radiculopathy is limited. Because capsaicin directly causes substance P release from neurons, it simultaneously induces pain while depleting the pain mediator and causing a dying-back phenomenon of nociceptive C-fibers in the dermis. The application of capsaicin can occur with a strong 1-time or 2-time application of 8% capsaicin or a slow graded increase in dose from 0.1% to 2.0% to allow for improved tolerability. The stronger doses may be less tolerated because of pain; however, a graded application requires frequent application for efficacy.[59] Thus, patient compliance is important for successful treatment.

Depending on the desired route of delivery, traditionally, oral medications can sometimes be compounded into a topical gel, cream, or ointment. Beyond the commercially available topical patches, a treatment compounded into a pluronic lecithin organogel or dimethyl sulfoxide carrier may have similar local or systemic effects of the medication. For instance, an anesthetic agent can be combined with an antispasticity medication for very specific local effects. Before prescribing, consideration should be given to the bioavailability, stability, and cost of topical treatments.

TREATMENT CONSIDERATIONS

The critical factor to consider is that there is no uniformly accepted treatment regimen for the treatment of painful lumbosacral radiculopathy. The pharmaceutical approach to the treatment should be individualized with an accompanying comprehensive exercise program to address the patient's specific pain complaint. Mild to moderate intermittent pain may be best handled with acetaminophen. Despite the lack of clear beneficial evidence as a category, NSAIDs may be used if there is an inflammatory component. However, the risk to benefit ratio of NSAIDs should be considered. This consideration is particularly true for those at increased risk of cardiovascular, GI, or renal adverse effects from NSAIDs. Muscle relaxants may be most helpful in the first few days of a radiculopathy but have few indications beyond that time period based on current evidence. The literature showing any efficacy for oral steroids in lumbosacral radiculopathy is limited.

Consideration should be given to the severity, chronicity, quality, and periodicity of pain complaints. If there is a physical movement that consistently decreases or eliminates a patient's pain complaints, this should be explored and treated if possible before prescribing a medication. When an analgesic is deemed necessary, the lowest dose with the fewest adverse effects should be used to achieve adequate pain relief. Analgesic medication should be given with consideration underlying medical conditions. These conditions may include hepatic or renal dysfunction, which may affect drug clearance. Similarly, it is also important to note conditions that may be worsened by drug administration, such as gastritis with NSAIDs. SNRIs and antiepileptic medications can be considered when neuropathic pain is present. Baseline and breakthrough pain should be addressed with appropriate dosing of long-acting and short-acting medications.

SUMMARY

Pharmacology for radiculopathy encompasses a variety of options ranging from the simple and effective, such as acetaminophen, to the complex manufactured molecules with limited evidence, such as tramadol. Neuromodulators likely play a significant role in mitigating neuropathic radicular symptoms. Consideration should be given to the role of medications in the context of the entire treatment plan, patient's comorbidities, drug-drug interactions, and ideal route of delivery.

REFERENCES

1. Chang V, Gonzalez P, Akuthota V. Evidence-informed management of chronic low back pain with adjunctive analgesics. Spine J 2008;8(1):21–7.
2. Chou R, Huffman LH. Medications for acute and chronic low back pain: a review of the evidence for an American Pain Society/American College of Physicians clinical practice guideline. Ann Intern Med 2007;147(7):505–14.
3. Haig AJ, Tomkins CC. Diagnosis and management of lumbar spinal stenosis. JAMA 2010;303(1):71.
4. Chou R. Pharmacological management of low back pain. Drugs 2010;70(4): 387–402.
5. Baron R, Freynhagen R, Tölle TR, et al. The efficacy and safety of pregabalin in the treatment of neuropathic pain associated with chronic lumbosacral radiculopathy. Pain 2010;150(3):420–7.
6. Devor M, Wall PD, Catalan N. Systemic lidocaine silences ectopic neuroma and DRG discharge without blocking nerve conduction. Pain 1992;48(2):261–8.
7. England JD, Happel LT, Kline DG, et al. Sodium channel accumulation in humans with painful neuromas. Neurology 1996;47(1):272–6.
8. Devor M, Seltzer Z. Pathophysiology of damaged nerves in relation to chronic pain. In: Wall PD, Melzack R, editors. Textbook of pain. Churchill Livingstone: Edinburgh; 1999. p.129–64.
9. Benzon H, Raja SN, Fishman SM, et al. Essentials of pain medicine and regional anesthesia. Philadelphia: Churchill Livingstone; 1999.

10. Towheed TE, Maxwell L, Judd MG, et al. Acetaminophen for osteoarthritis. Cochrane Database Syst Rev 2006;1:CD004257.
11. Zhang W, Jones A, Doherty M. Does paracetamol (acetaminophen) reduce the pain of osteoarthritis? A meta-analysis of randomised controlled trials. Ann Rheum Dis 2004;63(8):901–7.
12. Chou R, Qaseem A, Snow V, et al. Diagnosis and treatment of low back pain: a joint clinical practice guideline from the American College of Physicians and the American Pain Society. Ann Intern Med 2007;147(7):478–91.
13. McClain CJ, Price S, Barve S, et al. Acetaminophen hepatotoxicity: an update. Curr Gastroenterol Rep 1999;1(1):42–9.
14. Finnerup NB, Otto M, McQuay HJ, et al. Algorithm for neuropathic pain treatment: an evidence based proposal. Pain 2005;118(3):289–305.
15. Eisenberg E, McNicol ED, Carr DB. Efficacy and safety of opioid agonists in the treatment of neuropathic pain of nonmalignant origin: systematic review and meta-analysis of randomized controlled trials. JAMA 2005;293(24):3043.
16. Gilron I, Bailey JM, Tu D, et al. Morphine, gabapentin, or their combination for neuropathic pain. N Engl J Med 2005;352(13):1324.
17. Gatti A, Sabato AF, Occhioni R, et al. Controlled-release oxycodone and pregabalin in the treatment of neuropathic pain: results of a multicenter Italian study. Eur Neurol 2009;61(3):129–37.
18. Dworkin RH, O'Connor AB, Audette J, et al. Recommendations for the pharmacological management of neuropathic pain: an overview and literature update. Mayo Clin Proc 2010;85:S3–14.
19. Haanpää ML, Gourlay GK, Kent JL, et al. Treatment considerations for patients with neuropathic pain and other medical comorbidities. Mayo Clin Proc 2010; 85:S15–25.
20. Rhee JM, Schaufele M, Abdu WA. Radiculopathy and the herniated lumbar disc. Controversies regarding pathophysiology and management. J Bone Joint Surg Am 2006;88(9):2070.
21. McGeeney BE. Pharmacological management of neuropathic pain in older adults: an update on peripherally and centrally acting agents. J Pain Symptom Manage 2009;38(2):S15–27.
22. Dworkin RH, O'Connor AB, Backonja M, et al. Pharmacologic management of neuropathic pain: evidence-based recommendations. Pain 2007;132(3):237–51.
23. Cossman M, Wilsmann KM. Effect and side effects of tramadol: an open phase IV study with 7198 patients. Therapiewoche 1987;37:3475–85.
24. Pena M. Etodolac: analgesic effects in musculoskeletal and postoperative pain. Rheumatol Int 1990;10(Suppl):9–16.
25. Dreiser RL, Le Parc JM, Vélicitat P, et al. Oral meloxicam is effective in acute sciatica: two randomised, double-blind trials versus placebo or diclofenac. Inflamm Res 2001;50(Suppl 1):S17–23.
26. Lutz GE, Vad VB, Wisneski RJ. Fluoroscopic transforaminal lumbar epidural steroids: an outcome study. Arch Phys Med Rehabil 1998;79(11):1362–6.
27. Vad VB, Bhat AL, Lutz GE, et al. Transforaminal epidural steroid injections in lumbosacral radiculopathy: a prospective randomized study. Spine 2002;27(1): 11–6.
28. Saal J, Saal J, Yurth E. Nonoperative management of herniated cervical intervertebral disc with radiculopathy. Including commentary by Herzog RJ. Spine (Phila Pa 1976) 1996;21(16):1877–83.
29. Abram SE. Treatment of lumbosacral radiculopathy with epidural steroids. Anesthesiology 1999;91(6):1937.

30. Devor M, Govrin-Lippmann R, Raber P. Corticosteroids suppress ectopic neural discharge originating in experimental neuromas. Pain 1985;22(2):127–37.
31. Holve RL, Barkan H. Oral steroids in initial treatment of acute sciatica. J Am Board Fam Med 2008;21(5):469.
32. Finckh A, Zufferey P, Schurch MA, et al. Short-term efficacy of intravenous pulse glucocorticoids in acute discogenic sciatica. A randomized controlled trial. Spine 2006;31(4):377.
33. Haimovic IC, Beresford HR. Dexamethasone is not superior to placebo for treating lumbosacral radicular pain. Neurology 1986;36(12):1593.
34. Porsman O, Friis H. Prolapsed lumbar disc treated with intramuscularly administered dexamethasonephosphate: a prospectively planned, double-blind. Controlled clinical trial in 52 patients. Scand J Rheumatol 1979;8(3):142–4.
35. Nesbitt LT Jr. Minimizing complications from systemic glucocorticosteroid use. Dermatol Clin 1995;13(4):925.
36. Clark MR, Cox TS. Refractory chronic pain. Psychiatr Clin North Am 2002;25(1): 71–88.
37. Katon W, Egan K, Miller D. Chronic pain: lifetime psychiatric diagnoses and family history. Am J Psychiatry 1985;142(10):1156.
38. Fishbain DA, Goldberg M, Robert Meagher B, et al. Male and female chronic pain patients categorized by DSM-III psychiatric diagnostic criteria. Pain 1986;26(2): 181–97.
39. Evers AW, Kraaimaat FW, van Riel PL, et al. Cognitive, behavioral and physiological reactivity to pain as a predictor of long-term pain in rheumatoid arthritis patients. Pain 2001;93(2):139–46.
40. Harkins SW, Price DD, Braith J. Effects of extraversion and neuroticism on experimental pain, clinical pain, and illness behavior. Pain 1989;36(2):209–18.
41. Mossey JM, Gallagher RM, Tirumalasetti F. The effects of pain and depression on physical functioning in elderly residents of a continuing care retirement community. Pain Med 2000;1(4):340–50.
42. Preskorn SH, Greenblatt DJ, Flockhart D, et al. Comparison of duloxetine, escitalopram, and sertraline effects on cytochrome P450 2D6 function in healthy volunteers. J Clin Psychopharmacol 2007;27(1):28–34.
43. Fishbain DA, Cutler R, Rosomoff HL, et al. Evidence-based data from animal and human experimental studies on pain relief with antidepressants: a structured review. Pain Med 2000;1(4):310–6.
44. Thase ME, Entsuah AR, Rudolph RL. Remission rates during treatment with venlafaxine or selective serotonin reuptake inhibitors. Br J Psychiatry 2001;178(3):234.
45. Lovell J. Carbamazepine and sciatica. Aust Fam Physician 1992;21(6):784.
46. Yildirim K, Sisecioglu M, Karatay S, et al. The effectiveness of gabapentin in patients with chronic radiculopathy. Pain Clinic 2003;15(3):213–8.
47. Saldaña MT, Navarro A, Pérez C, et al. A cost-consequences analysis of the effect of pregabalin in the treatment of painful radiculopathy under medical practice conditions in primary care settings. Pain Pract 2010;10(1):31–41.
48. Khoromi S, Patsalides A, Parada S, et al. Topiramate in chronic lumbar radicular pain. J Pain 2005;6(12):829–36.
49. Muehlbacher M, Nickel MK, Kettler C, et al. Topiramate in treatment of patients with chronic low back pain: a randomized, double-blind, placebo-controlled study. Clin J Pain 2006;22(6):526.
50. Eisenberg E, Damunni G, Hoffer E, et al. Lamotrigine for intractable sciatica: correlation between dose, plasma concentration and analgesia. Eur J Pain 2003;7(6):485–91.

51. Hamza MS, Anderson DG, Snyder JW, et al. Effectiveness of levetiracetam in the treatment of lumbar radiculopathy: an open-label prospective cohort study. PM R 2009;1(4):335–9.
52. Serpell MG. Gabapentin in neuropathic pain syndromes: a randomised, double-blind, placebo-controlled trial. Pain 2002;99(3):557–66.
53. Semenchuk MR, Sherman S. Effectiveness of tizanidine in neuropathic pain: an open-label study. J Pain 2000;1(4):285–92.
54. Browning R, Jackson JL, O'Malley PG. Cyclobenzaprine and back pain: a meta-analysis. Arch Intern Med 2001;161(13):1613–20.
55. Asiedu M, Ossipov MH, Kaila K, et al. Acetazolamide and midazolam act synergistically to inhibit neuropathic pain. Pain 2010;148(2):302–8.
56. Chou R, Peterson K, Helfand M. Comparative efficacy and safety of skeletal muscle relaxants for spasticity and musculoskeletal conditions: a systematic review. J Pain Symptom Manage 2004;28(2):140–75.
57. Goupille P, Mulleman D, Valat J. Radiculopathy associated with disc herniation. Ann Rheum Dis 2006;65(2):141–3.
58. Korhonen T, Karppinen J, Paimela L, et al. The treatment of disc herniation-induced sciatica with infliximab: one-year follow-up results of FIRST II, a randomized controlled trial. Spine 2006;31(24):2759.
59. Watson CP. Topical capsaicin as an adjuvant analgesic. J Pain Symptom Manage 1994;9(7):425–33.

The Efficacy of Lumbar Epidural Steroid Injections: Transforaminal, Interlaminar, and Caudal Approaches

Monica E. Rho, MD[a],*, Chi-Tsai Tang, MD[b]

KEYWORDS

• Low back pain • Epidural steroid injection • Efficacy
• Transforaminal • Interlaminar • Caudal

The effectiveness of lumbosacral epidural corticosteroid injections has often been studied in the literature; however, it has been difficult to summarize because of the wide variability of study designs used to demonstrate efficacy. There are also multiple approaches to reach the lumbar epidural space (transforaminal, interlaminar, and caudal approaches), which further complicate the issue of determining which injection is the most efficacious. There are only a few randomized controlled trials that compared a lumbar transforaminal epidural steroid injection (TFESI) to a placebo control. Complicating the issue even more is that there is no standard placebo control for this type of study. The placebo interventions have ranged from paraspinal saline trigger point injections to transforaminal injections (TFIs) with local anesthetic or saline. However, it is debatable whether a TFI with saline is a true placebo, because there have been studies demonstrating the therapeutic effect of a saline epidural injection.[1,2] Interlaminar epidural steroid injections (ILESIs) and caudal epidural steroid injections (ESIs) have been used for a longer period, but given the recent trend of

---

No funding or support was provided in the writing of this article.

The authors have nothing to disclose.

[a] Department of Physical Medicine and Rehabilitation, Northwestern University Feinberg School of Medicine/Rehabilitation Institute of Chicago, 345 East Superior Street, Chicago, IL 60611, USA

[b] Department of Orthopaedic Surgery, Division of Physical Medicine and Rehabilitation, Washington University School of Medicine, Washington University Orthopedics, One Barnes--Jewish Hospital Plaza, Suite 11300, Campus Box 8233, St Louis, MO 63110, USA

* Corresponding author.

E-mail address: mrho@ric.org

Phys Med Rehabil Clin N Am 22 (2011) 139–148

doi:10.1016/j.pmr.2010.10.006

1047-9651/11/$ – see front matter © 2011 Elsevier Inc. All rights reserved.

TFESIs, studies comparing ILESIs and caudal injections with placebo are rare. Further complicating the issue, the number of injections used for each study, the type of corticosteroid used, the volume of injectate, the inclusion and exclusion criteria of the participants, and the outcome measures vary across all studies. Determining a consensus statement on the efficacy of lumbar ESIs is extremely difficult for this reason, and many meta-analyses and systematic reviews on this topic have produced conflicting results.[3–12] This article presents the data on the efficacy of lumbosacral epidural corticosteroid injections organized by levels of evidence based on criteria set by Wright in 2005 (**Table 1**).[13] This is not a systematic review, and the studies described are merely a representation of the strongest study designs and most-frequently referenced studies on the efficacy of lumbar ESIs.

LEVEL 1 EVIDENCE
Efficacy of Steroids in TFESI

One of the most frequently cited studies comes from Riew and colleagues[14] in 2000. A total of 55 patients with unilateral lumbar radicular pain and radiographically confirmed herniated nucleus pulposus (HNP) or spinal stenosis were enrolled. Every patient was considered a surgical candidate by the patient and the surgeon. These patients were randomized into a group with 1 to 4 TFIs with bupivacaine (n = 27) versus a group with 1 to 4 TFESIs with bupivacaine and betamethasone (n = 28). Both the subjects and the treating surgeon were blinded to the intervention. Follow-up occurred at 13 to 28 months postinjection, and 67% of patients in the control group went on to have surgery, whereas only 29% of the treatment group pursued surgical intervention. This difference was statistically significant ($P<.004$). These results present strong evidence that in surgical candidates with radicular pain secondary to HNP or spinal stenosis, a TFESI is a surgery-sparring intervention compared with TFI of bupivacaine alone.

In 2006, Riew and colleagues[15] followed up on all the patients who avoided surgery in the initial study. There were 29 patients who avoided surgery in the first 28 months post-injection, of which 9 were in the control group and 20 were in the treatment group.

Table 1	
Levels of evidence for therapeutic studies	
Levels of Evidence	**Criteria**

Level 1	Randomized controlled trials
	  With a significant difference
	  With no significant difference but narrow confidence intervals
	Systematic review of level 1 randomized controlled trials

Level 2	Prospective cohort study
	Randomized controlled trials
	  Poor quality (eg, <80% follow-up, low power, poor randomization
	    technique, unblinded evaluators)
	Systematic review
	  Level 2 studies
	  Nonhomogeneous level 1 studies

Level 3	Case-control study Retrospective cohort study Systematic review of level 3 studies
Level 4	Case series
Level 5	Expert opinion

Eight patients in the treatment group were lost to follow-up. Of those who initially avoided surgery in 2000, 8 of 9 in the control group and 9 of 12 in the treatment group still had not had surgery at the 5-year follow-up. The difference between the groups was not statistically significant, which suggests that TFESIs do not make a significant difference in the long-term outcome when it comes to pursuing surgery, although all patients lost to follow-up were in the treatment group.

In 2001, Karppinen and colleagues[16] used a single saline TFI as the placebo (n = 80) against a single TFESI with methylprednisolone and bupivacaine (n = 80). There were 160 patients who reported unilateral leg pain greater than back pain for 3 to 28 weeks. The patients were randomized and the intervention was double blinded. Outcome measures included back visual analog scale (VAS), leg VAS, Oswestry Low Back Disability Questionnaire, Nottingham Health Profile, cost, and physical examination maneuvers (straight leg raise, modified Schober measure, muscle strength testing, sensation testing, and reflexes). A single injection was given to each patient. Immediately after the injection, leg pain decreased by 61% in the treatment group and by 44% in the control group. At 2 weeks post-injection, there were statistically significant improvements in all measures (except the Schober measure) for both groups. At 3 months, the control group had a greater reduction in back pain than the treatment group. At 6 months, the control group had a greater reduction in both back and leg pain than the treatment group. At 1-year follow-up, both groups demonstrated statistically significant improvements compared with their status before injections, but there were no between-group differences. In addition, 23% of the treatment group and 19% of the control group went on to pursue a surgical intervention. The study concluded that the combination of methylprednisolone and bupivacaine in a TFESI seemed to have a short-term effect in both subjective and objective improvement of pain, but the effect did not last longer than 3 months post-injection.

Using the same 160 patients, Karppinen and colleagues[17] published an in-depth subgroup analysis of the outcomes from the original study. They looked at contained HNP versus disc extrusions. In contained herniations, the treatment group (methylprednisolone and bupivacaine TFESI) had significantly improved leg pain at 2 and 4 weeks postinjection compared with the control group (saline TFI). The same trend was not seen in the disc extrusion subgroup. This study also concluded that patients receiving steroid treatment of a contained herniation were less likely to undergo back surgery and they also had significantly fewer days on sick leave at 3 to 6 months postinjection. There were also significant medical cost savings as early as 4 weeks postinjection and for as long as 1 year postinjection. In contrast, patients with disc extrusions who received the saline injection tended to have less cumulative medical costs after 3 and 12 months than those given the steroid injection, suggesting that a steroid injection seemed to be more harmful for disc extrusions, based on the hypothesis that macrophages are more prominent in disc extrusions and play a role in resorption that is disrupted by the introduction of steroids. Within the disc extrusion group, there were significantly more subjects who required surgical intervention after 10 weeks postinjection. The administration of steroids seems to be countereffective in the disc extrusion group.

Ng and colleagues[18] studied 86 subjects with chronic unilateral radicular pain from HNP or foraminal stenosis that failed conservative treatment. The control group received a single TFI with bupivacaine only (n = 43), and the treatment group received a single TFESI with bupivacaine and methylprednisolone (n = 43). The outcomes were assessed at 6 and 12 weeks postinjection. The study found improvement in both groups for leg pain, Oswestry score, and walking distances, with no significant differences between the 2 groups. Only the duration of symptoms demonstrated a statistically significant predictive response. The shorter the duration of symptoms, the better the outcomes of the injection in both the control and treatment groups.

In 2010, Ghahreman and colleagues[19] conducted a study on 150 patients who had pain radiating in the lower limb with a positive straight leg raise (SLR) and a disc herniation confirmed by computed tomography (CT) or magnetic resonance imaging (MRI). The subjects where then randomized into receiving a fluoroscopically-guided lumbar TFI of a steroid (triamcinolone), a local anesthetic (bupivacaine) or saline versus a placebo intramuscular injection of steroid or saline. If patients did not respond to the initial injection, they were allowed additional injections up to 3 total injections. The primary outcome measure was the proportion of patients who obtained complete relief or at least 50% relief of pain for at least 1 month after treatment. Results demonstrated that there was a significantly greater proportion of subjects treated with a TFESI (54%) who achieved relief of pain when compared with patients treated with TFI of local anesthetic (7%) or saline (19%) or intramuscular injections of steroids (21%) or saline (13%). Relief of pain was accompanied by significant improvements in function and disability. Over time, the relief of pain diminished in all groups equally.

Efficacy of TFESI Versus ILESI Versus Caudal ESI

Not all level 1 studies used a placebo as a control. In 2007, Ackerman and Ahmad[20] compared the 3 different approaches to the epidural space (TFESI, ILESI, and caudal ESI). There were 90 subjects with L5-S1 disc herniations on imaging and severe S1 radicular pain confirmed as S1 radiculopathy by electromyography. The subjects were evenly randomized into each treatment group, and they all received the same dose of triamcinolone and saline. The same injection was given every 2 weeks for a total of 3 injections if adequate pain relief was not achieved. On average, subjects in the TFESI group received 1.5 injections, the ILESI group received 2.2 injections, and the caudal group received 2.5 injections. At 2 weeks postinjection, pain scores were reduced in all 3 groups; however, the TFESI group had a significantly greater reduction. Oswestry and Beck depression scores improved in all 3 groups without any between-group differences. There were also significantly more cases of complete pain relief in patients who had a ventral dispersion pattern of contrast flow, a flow pattern that occurred more consistently with the TFESI group. This study suggests that a transforaminal approach offers the benefit of increased analgesic efficacy, possibly because of an increased ventral spread of the steroid solution in the case of a herniated or extruded disc.

Efficacy of ILESI Versus Discectomy

In 2004, Buttermann[21] looked at surgical outcomes versus conservative care in a patient population with a large HNP. A total of 100 patients who had no improvement after a minimum of 6 weeks of noninvasive care were followed for a 3-year period. They were randomly assigned to either receive an ILESI or have a discectomy. Those in the ILESI group were given repeated injections administered 1 week apart up to a maximum of 3 injections if needed. About 76% of the patients in the ILESI group received fluoroscopically-guided injections. Follow-up was performed at 1–3, 4–6, and 7–12 months and at 1–2 and 2–3 years after treatment. There was a crossover group of 27 patients who considered ILESI treatment a failure and subsequently went on to discectomy. The results demonstrated that the discectomy group had earlier motor recovery than the ESI group. Fewer patients in the discectomy group had a motor deficit at 1–3 months posttreatment ($P = .001$). However, at the 2–3 year follow-up, there were no significant differences between the 2 groups in regard to motor weakness. Both groups demonstrated a significant decrease in both back and lower extremity pain VAS scores compared with pretreatment levels; however, the decrease in lower extremity pain scores in the discectomy group was significantly greater than in the ILESI group at the 1–3 month and 4–6 month follow-up intervals. Functional outcome improved significantly in both groups at all follow-up intervals. This study supported the use of ILESI in patients with continued severe symptoms after 6 weeks of noninvasive treatment because nearly half of these patients who received the ESI had a fairly rapid decrease in their symptoms without requiring surgery. The degree of improvement was similar to that for those who underwent a discectomy. Those who failed the ESI and went on to have the discectomy also demonstrated the same decline in pain scores and improvement in functional outcome scores despite the delay of surgery by at least 1 month. The delay to surgery did not seem to adversely affect the overall outcome for the patient.

Efficacy of Steroids in Non-guided ILESI

In 1997, Carette and colleagues[22] examined nonguided ILESI as a means to treat sciatica caused by HNP. In this randomized, double-blind trial, there were 156 patients with intermittent pain in one or both legs, with a minimum duration of 4 weeks and a maximum duration of 1 year. They also had signs of nerve root irritation (positive SLR) or nerve root compression (motor, sensory, or reflex deficits). All patients had evidence of HNP by CT scan. Patients were randomized to receive either 2 mL of methylprednisolone mixed with 8 mL of saline or 1 mL of saline into the epidural space. All injections were non-guided, and repeat injections were done after 3 and 6 weeks if the patient did not report a marked improvement in their symptoms. At 3 weeks post-injection, the ILESI group demonstrated improvements in spine mobility and sensory deficits compared with the placebo group. At 6 weeks, there was more improvement in leg pain in the ILESI group. After 3 months, there were no significant differences between the groups. After 1 year, both groups had similar surgical rates (ILESI group, 25.8% and placebo group, 24.8%). Overall, non-guided ILESI demonstrated short-term improvements in radicular pain and spinal mobility compared with an interlaminar epidural injection of saline. There were no long-term differences seen between both the groups.

In 2003, Valat and colleagues[23] also examined the efficacy of steroids in non-guided ILESI. Eighty-eight patients with unilateral sciatica lasting 15 to 180 days were randomized to receive 3 non-guided interlaminar epidural injections at 2-day intervals with either 2 mL of prednisolone (n = 39) or 2 mL of isotonic saline (n = 35). Self-assessment at day 20 was the outcome measure. On analysis, 12 of 35 (34%) in the control group and 22 of 39 (56%) in the steroid group had successful pain relief, but this result was not statistically significant between groups. The investigators concluded that ESI provided no additional improvement compared with isotonic saline when administered using a non-guided interlaminar approach. This outcome differs from that observed by Carette and colleagues[22]; however, a different volume of injectate (2 mL) was used in the 2 studies (2 mL Valat[23]; 10 mL Carette[22]).

Efficacy of Steroids in Caudal ESI

Although caudal ESIs have been around the longest, there are not many randomized controlled trials published recently on this topic. The most recent study was done by Sayegh and colleagues[24] in 2009. They looked at 183 patients with severe chronic low back pain and sciatica. The patients were randomized into 2 groups. Both the groups were given a non-guided caudal epidural injection; group A was given Xylocaine and betamethasone (n = 93), and group B was given Xylocaine and water (n = 90). The investigators found that the steroid group experienced faster relief at the 1-week post-injection follow-up and had significant functional improvements on the Oswestry scores at all follow-up visits. SLR improved in both groups after the injection but improved earlier for the group given the betamethasone. This study concluded that a caudal epidural injection containing local anesthetic and steroids or water seems to be effective in treating patient with low back pain and sciatica; however, those receiving the steroid preparation demonstrated better and faster efficacy from the injection.

LEVEL 2 EVIDENCE
Efficacy of TFESI

In 2002, Vad and colleagues[25] compared TFESI to paraspinal saline trigger point injections. This study was completed on 48 patients with MRI evidence of HNP with less than 50% intervertebral foraminal narrowing who reported leg pain greater than back pain, with symptoms lasting more than 6 weeks. The controls were given 1 to 2 paraspinal trigger point injections of saline, and the intervention group received 1 to 3 TFESIs of Xylocaine and betamethasone. The investigators defined a successful outcome as a satisfaction score of 2 (good) or 3 (very good), improvement on the Roland-Morris score of 5 or more, and pain reduction greater than 50% at least 1 year after treatment. After an average follow-up of 1.4 years, the TFESI group had a success rate of 84% compared with the 48% success rate of the control group ($P<.005$). The main limitation of this study was that the patients and researchers were not blinded to the treatment; however, the study strongly suggests that in the setting of radicular pain caused by HNP lasting longer than 6 weeks, a TFESI improves symptoms and patient satisfaction more than trigger point injections into the paraspinal muscles.

Most of the studies on this subject focus on a surgically naive patient population. In 1999, Devulder and colleagues[26] sought to evaluate the outcome of TFI in patients with failed back surgery syndrome. They looked at 60 postsurgical patients with documented nerve fibrosis on epidurogram and MRI as well as electromyogram-confirmed chronic nerve pathology without acute irritation. Using a transforaminal approach, a selective epidural nerve root sleeve injection was performed under fluoroscopy. The patients were randomized into 1 of 3 groups. Group A was given a solution of bupivacaine, hyaluronidase, and saline (n = 20). Group B was given bupivacaine and methylprednisolone (n = 20). Group C was given bupivacaine, hyaluronidase, and methylprednisolone (n = 20). All injections were of equal volume, and all patients received a total of 2 injections of the same solution, separated by a 1-week interval. All 3 groups demonstrated pain relief after the first month and a decline in pain relief at 3 and 6 months postinjection. Overall, there were no statistically significant differences in pain relief among the 3 groups. This study suggests that in patients with chronic failed back surgery syndrome, there is no improvement in pain scores after a TFESI or a TFI of bupivacaine, hyaluronidase, and saline.

Efficacy of TFESI Versus ILESI

There are a few studies that compared TFESI with ILESI directly. Kolsi and colleagues[27] studied 30 patients with severe radicular pain, positive SLR, and imaging findings consistent with HNP. The subjects were randomized to a single fluoroscopically guided ILESI (n = 13) or a single fluoroscopically guided TFESI (n = 17). Both groups were given the same dose of lidocaine and cortivazol. VAS for leg and low back pain, percent improvement score, analgesic use, Schober test, finger-to-floor distance with lumbar flexion, and an EIFEL score were used as outcome measures and were taken pre-injection and at days 1, 7, 14, 21 and 28 post-injection. There were no statistically significant differences between both the groups in regard to these outcome measures. Another follow-up was done verbally at a mean of 8 months post-injection. At that time, 3 of 17 patients in the TFESI group and 3 of 13 patients in the ILESI group had pursued surgical intervention for their symptoms; this was not a significant difference. This study is limited because of its small sample size, but it concludes that there are no differences in outcome between TFESI and ILESI in patients with radicular pain caused by HNP.

In 2002, Thomas and colleagues[28] also tried to compare TFESI with ILESI, using dexamethasone for both injections. Thirty-one patients who were hospitalized for acute radicular pain lasting for less than 3 months with HNP on imaging were recruited into the study. Sixteen patients were randomized to receive a non-guided ILESI, and 15 patients were randomized to receive a fluoroscopically-guided TFESI. The results demonstrated that the TFESI group had improvement in the Schober test, finger-to-floor distance with lumbar flexion, and Dallas scores on day 6. They had improved VAS scores at day 30 and superior VAS scores, Roland-Morris scores, and Dallas scores when compared with the ILESI group at 6 months post-injection. Thomas and colleagues concluded that TFESI provided superior pain relief and functional improvement when compared with non-guided ILESI in patients hospitalized for acute radicular pain.

In 2008, Candido and colleagues[29] compared TFESI with ILESI using a parasagittal interlaminar approach under fluoroscopic-guidance. The investigators postulate that using the parasagittal interlaminar approach makes it more likely for the injectate to spread to the anterior epidural space, which is closer to the nerve root/intervertebral disc interface, thus potentially having a greater effect without the risks of a TFESI. Fifty-seven patients with low back pain and unilateral radiculopathy with radiographic evidence of HNP, degenerative disc disease, or spinal stenosis were enrolled in the study. Subjects were randomly assigned to the TFESI group (n = 28) or the parasagittal ILESI group (n = 29). Both groups were given the same injectate (methylprednisolone, lidocaine, and saline). The results demonstrated equal contrast flow patterns, and the parasagittal interlaminar approach was able to achieve anterior epidural flow 100% of the time. There was a significantly reduced (P = .003) mean fluoroscopic time in the ILESI group (28.96 seconds) when compared with the TFESI group (46.25 seconds). VAS scores were equivalent between groups throughout the follow-up period. Candido and colleagues concluded that a parasagittal interlaminar approach under fluoroscopic-guidance should be used in patients with radicular low back pain caused by HNP, degenerative disc disease, or spinal stenosis, because there was less overall exposure to radiation, similar improvement in VAS scores, and less overall risk with this approach in comparison to a TFESI.

LEVEL 3 EVIDENCE

In 2006, Schaufele and colleagues[30] designed a case-control study which retrospectively identified 40 patients who received their first fluoroscopically-guided ESI for radicular pain caused by HNP. Twenty patients received a TFESI, and 20 patients had an ILESI. There was a significant improvement in the pain scores in both groups immediately after injection and at follow-up, which occurred at an average of 17.1 days postinjection; however, the TFESI resulted in better short-term pain improvement and demonstrated fewer long-term surgical interventions than the ILESI group.

Manchikanti and colleagues[31] compared the 3 routes of ESIs in a retrospective evaluation of 225 patients with chronic low back pain. The 3 groups were (1) nonguided ILESI, (2) caudal ESI, and (3) fluoroscopy-guided TFESI. All the 3 approaches were effective in obtaining relief for the patients, although the caudal and transforaminal approaches were the most successful in obtaining longer-term relief. The TFESI group obtained the greatest relief with the least medical expenses.

LEVEL 4 EVIDENCE

Level 4 evidence is clearly not as strong as the other evidences provided; however, there is one prospective case series that really brought attention to TFESIs and encouraged the development of higher-level studies to compare the efficacy of TFESI with that of the previously more common approach to the lumbar epidural space. Lutz and colleagues[32] published a prospective case series on patients with lumbar HNP and radiculopathy who received a TFESI. Sixty-nine patients were followed up from 28 to 144 weeks. About 75.4% of the patients had a successful long-term outcome, reporting at least a 50% or more reduction between preinjection and postinjection pain scores. Patients were able to return to or near their previous level of function after only 1.8 injections per patient, and 78.3% of patients were satisfied with their final outcome.

SUMMARY OF THE EVIDENCE AND INDICATIONS FOR INJECTIONS

There is strong evidence to support the use of lumbar TFESI in patients with acute to subacute unilateral radicular pain caused by HNP or spinal stenosis.[15,16,18,19,25] There is no relief of pain with a TFESI in patients with chronic failed back surgery syndrome and documented fibrosis of the nerves.[26] The greatest relief of pain occurs in the leg.[19] There is insufficient evidence to support the use of ESI for axial discogenic low back pain. The effect of the injection seems to work best in the short term and does not necessarily give long-term effects.[16,18] A lumbar TFESI is an effective surgery-sparing procedure that should be a part of conservative care in the management of low back pain with radiculopathy.[15] It was also found that delaying surgery in patients with a large herniated disc to attempt ILESI did not change the surgical outcomes of those who failed the injections.[21] In fact, approximately 50% of those patients who delayed surgery to attempt the ILESI did not require surgery. It was also demonstrated that the degree of pain relief from the ILESI matched the surgical outcome scores after discectomy.[21]

Although there is evidence that demonstrates the short-term efficacy of ILESI and caudal epidural injections in the management of low back and radicular pain,[20–22,24] when compared head-to-head with TFESI, the greatest pain relief and the lowest average number of injections to achieve pain relief occurs with TFESI.[20,28] The rationale of improved pain scores with TFESI is made by observed contrast flow patterns. The transforaminal approach demonstrates more ventral epidural flow, which is where most of the pathologic changes occur. One study attempted to mimic the ventral epidural flow pattern by adjusting the interlaminar approach technique. By using a more parasagittal interlaminar approach, a better ventral epidural flow was achieved, which resulted in improved pain scores after a parasagittal ILESI when compared with the standard TFESI.[29] The parasagittal ILESI required fluoroscopic guidance. Nonguided ILESI showed short-term improvement in pain, mobility, and functional outcome in at least one study[22] but did not demonstrate any statistically significant improvement compared with an interlaminar epidural injection with saline in another study.[23] It is recommended to perform all ESIs under fluoroscopic guidance.

There is at least one study comparing fluoroscopically-guided TFESI with ILESI that did not demonstrate significant differences in outcomes between the 2 groups; however, all subjects were limited to a single injection.[27] Most of the evidence suggests that although some patients improve after 1 injection, other patients will likely need repeated injections to receive improved pain relief. The intervals between injections varied between 2 days and 2 weeks (the authors recommend 2 weeks), and the maximum number of injections varied between 3 and 4 injections.

Lumbar ESIs can be an effective tool in the conservative management of low back pain with radicular symptoms. These injections should not be used as first-line treatment but, rather, in conjunction with conservative therapy and oral medications. These injections are invasive procedures that do not come without risks and potential complications. Selecting the best approach to the epidural space for each patient and using fluoroscopic-guidance during the procedure limits the risk and complications. Properly trained and experienced physicians should be performing these procedures to ensure maximal safety and efficacy for the patient.

REFERENCES

1. Bhatia MT, Parikh CJ. Epidural-saline therapy in lumbosciatic syndrome. J Indian Med Assoc 1966;47:537–42.
2. Gupta AK, Mital VK, Azmi RU. Observations on the management of lumbosciatic syndrome (sciatica) by epidural saline injection. J Indian Med Assoc 1970;54:194–6.
3. Nelemans PJ, deBie RA, deVe HC, et al. Injection therapy for subacute and chronic benign low back pain [review]. Spine 2001;26:501–15.
4. Roberts ST, Willick SE, Rho ME, et al. Efficacy of lumbosacral transforaminal epidural steroid injections: a systematic review. PM R 2009;1:657–68.
5. Boswell MV, Hansen HC, Trescot AM, et al. Epidural steroids in the management of chronic spinal pain and radiculopathy. Pain Physician 2003;6:319–34.
6. DePalma MJ, Bhargava A, Slipman CW. A critical appraisal of the evidence for selective nerve root injection in the treatment of lumbosacral radiculopathy. Arch Phys Med Rehabil 2005;86:1477–83.
7. Young IA, Hyman GS, Packia-Raj LN, et al. The use of lumbar epidural/transforaminal steroids for managing spinal disease. J Am Acad Orthop Surg 2007;15:228–38.
8. Abdi S, Datta S, Trescot AM, et al. Epidural steroids in the management of chronic spinal pain: A systematic review. Pain Physician 2007;10:185–212.
9. Armon C, Argoff CE, Samuels J, et al. Assessment: use of epidural steroid injections to treat radicular lumbosacral pain: report of the Therapeutics and Technology Assessment Subcommittee of the American Academy of Neurology. Neurology 2007;68:723–9.
10. Buenaventura RM, Datta S, Abdi S, et al. Systematic review of therapeutic lumbar transforaminal epidural steroid injections. Pain Physician 2009;12:233–51.
11. Levin JH. Prospective, double-blind, randomized placebo-controlled trials in interventional spine: what the highest quality literature tells us. Spine J 2009;9: 690–703.
12. McLain RF, Kapural L, Mekhail NA. Epidural steroid therapy for back and leg pain: mechanisms of action and efficacy. Spine J 2005;5:191–201.
13. Wright JG. Introducing levels of evidence to the journal. JBJS 2003;85A(1):1–3.
14. Riew KD, Yin Y, Gilula L, et al. The effect of nerve-root injections on the need for operative treatment of lumbar radicular pain. A prospective, randomized, controlled, double-blind study. J Bone Joint Surg Am 2000;82-A:1589–93.
15. Riew KD, Park JB, Cho YS, et al. Nerve root blocks in the treatment of lumbar radicular pain. A minimum five-year follow-up. J Bone Joint Surg Am 2006; 88(8):1722–5.

16. Karppinen J, Malmivaara A, Kurunlahti M, et al. Periradicular infiltration for sciatica: a randomized controlled trial. Spine 2001;26:1059–67.
17. Karppinen J, Ohinmaa A, Malmivaara A, et al. Cost effectiveness of periradicular infiltration for sciatica: subgroup analysis of a randomized controlled trial. Spine 2001;26(23):2587–95.
18. Ng L, Chaudhary N, Sell P. The efficacy of corticosteroids in periradicular infiltration for chronic radicular pain: a randomized, double blind, controlled trial. Spine 2005;30:857–62.
19. Ghahreman A, Ferch R, Bogduk N. The efficacy of transforaminal injection of steroids for the treatment of lumbar radicular pain. Pain Med 2010;11:1149–68.
20. Ackermann WE, Ahmad M. The efficacy of lumbar epidural steroid injections in patients with lumbar disc herniations. Anesth Analg 2007;104:1217–22.
21. Buttermann GR. Treatment of lumbar disc herniation: epidural steroid injection compared with discectomy. J Bone Joint Surg Am 2004;86(4):670–9.
22. Carette S, Leclaire R, Marcoux S, et al. Epidural corticosteroid injections for sciatica due to herniated nucleus pulposus. N Engl J Med 1997;336(23):1634–40.
23. Valat JP, Giraudau B, Rozenberg S, et al. Epidural corticosteroid injections for sciatica: a randomized, double-blind, controlled clinical trial. Ann Rheum Dis 2003;62:639–43.
24. Sayegh FE, Kenanidis EI, Papavasiliou KA, et al. Efficacy of steroid and nonsteroid caudal epidural injections for low back pain and sciatica: a prospective, randomized, double-blind clinical trial. Spine 2009;34:1441–7.
25. Vad VB, Bhat AL, Lutz GE, et al. Transforaminal epidural steroid injections in lumbosacral radiculopathy: a prospective randomized study. Spine 2002;27:11–6.
26. Devulder J, Deene P, DeLaat M, et al. Nerve root sleeve injections in patients with failed back surgery syndrome: a comparison of three solutions. Clin J Pain 1999; 15(2):132–5.
27. Kolsi I, Delecrin J, Berthelot JM, et al. Efficacy of nerve root versus interspinous injections of glucocorticoids in the treatment of disk-related sciatica. A pilot, prospective randomized, double-blind study. Joint Bone Spine 2000;67:113–8.
28. Thomas E, Cyteval C, Abiad L, et al. Efficacy of transforaminal versus interspinous corticosteroid injection in discal radicalgia – a prospective randomized, double-blind study. Clin Rheumatol 2003;22:299–304.
29. Candido KD, Raghavendra MS, Chinthagada M, et al. A prospective evaluation of iodinated contrast flow patterns with fluoroscopically guided lumbar epidural steroid injections: the lateral parasagittal interlaminar epidural approach versus the transforaminal epidural approach. Anesth Analg 2008;106(2):638–44.
30. Schaufele MK, Hatch L, Jones W. Interlaminar versus transforaminal epidural injections for the treatment of symptomatic lumbar intervertebral disc herniations. Pain Physician 2006;9:361–6.
31. Manchikanti L, Pakanati RR, Pampati V. Comparison of three routes of epidural steroid injections in low back pain. Pain Digest 1999;9:277–85.
32. Lutz GE, Vad VB, Wisneski RJ. Fluoroscopic transforaminal lumbar epidural steroids: an outcome study. Arch Phys Med Rehabil 1998;79:1362–6.

Epidural Steroid Injections for Cervical Radiculopathy

Alison Stout, DO[a,b,*]

KEYWORDS

- Epidural steroid • Spine intervention • Cervical
- Radiculopathy • Transforaminal • Interlaminar • Treatment

The injection of glucocorticoid (steroid) medication into the epidural space to treat back pain was first performed in the 1950s.[1] The first publication of cervical epidural steroid injection (ESI) for radicular pain was in 1961.[2] In the 1960s, initial reports in the United States described treatment of sciatica using the caudal and interlaminar (IL) approaches.[3,4] By the mid 1970s, injections via the transforaminal (TF) approach alongside the nerve root were described in combination with fluoroscopic radiograph guidance.

The founding principle of injecting steroid and anesthetic medication into the epidural space is that it decreases pain and inflammation at the site of injection. A herniated disc is the most commonly proposed mechanism of increased inflammation and pain. Herniated disc material has been shown to cause an inflammatory response in the dura, nerve roots, dorsal root ganglion, and the spinal cord, with a notable increase of phospholipase A_2 activity.[5] Human lumbar disc herniation extracts have shown 20 to 10,000 times greater phospholipase A_2 activity than any other human source.[5] Other immunohistochemical substances implicated in increasing inflammation and pain from discs include matrix nitric oxide, metalloproteinases, prostaglandin E_2, and interleukin 6.[6,7] The hypothesis is that steroid medication in the epidural space interrupts the inflammatory cascade in addition to inhibiting neural transmission by nociceptive C fibers. Disc herniation is only one possible cause, and cervical spondylotic foraminal and central stenosis can also cause radiculopathy. The various etiologies of radiculopathy may respond differently to ESIs.

[a] Rehabilitation Care Services, Veterans Administration, Puget Sound, 117-RCS, 1660 South Columbian Way, Seattle, WA 98108, USA
[b] Department of Rehabilitation, University of Washington, Seattle, WA 98195, USA
* Corresponding author. Rehabilitation Care Services, Veterans Administration, Puget Sound, 117-RCS, 1660 South Columbian Way, Seattle, WA 98108.
E-mail address: stouta@uw.edu

Phys Med Rehabil Clin N Am 22 (2011) 149–159
doi:10.1016/j.pmr.2010.10.007
1047-9651/11/$ – see front matter. Published by Elsevier Inc.

pmr.theclinics.com

GENERAL INDICATIONS

ESIs have been used to treat a variety of spinal disorders. They are primarily and most widely accepted as a treatment of radicular symptoms. Patients with radicular pain that has been unresponsive to noninterventional care for 1 to 2 months including physical therapy, medications, and education are candidates for ESIs. In patients without progressive neurologic deficit or cervical myelopathy, ESIs are considered as a rational part of treatment before surgical intervention. However, the potential benefits must be weighed against the possible risks for each patient.

COMPLICATIONS OF ESIs

In general, risks of spine interventions are related to needle placement, the medications used, and patient factors. These include, but are not limited to, tissue trauma, bleeding, infection, nerve/cord injury, spinal block, medication side effects/toxicity, and allergic reaction. Minor procedural complications vasovagal reactions, nausea, transient neurologic symptoms, and increased neck or arm pain. Transient complications with ESIs can occur as a result of side effects of steroids, anesthetics, and contrast dye. Another risk to consider is radiation exposure. More specific risks for cervical ESIs depend on the route of administration. Both the IL and the TF routes have risk, but the TF route has a higher rate of major complications.

A recent review of cervical IL ESI complications included studies from 1996 to 2005.[8] The investigators cited 2 studies specific to IL ESI, one documenting the rate of complication as just less than 1%, whereas conversely the other reported a 16.8% rate. Minor complications included increased axial neck pain, nonpositional headache, facial flushing, vasovagal episode, superficial skin infection at the site of injection, insomnia, and nausea/vomiting. Major complications included epidural hematoma, subdural hematoma, subdural block, intrathecal block, dural puncture, persistent/permanent neuropathic symptoms, intracranial hypotension and granuloma, permanent spinal cord injury, pneumocephalus, venous air embolism, cervical epidural abscess, and Cushing syndrome for 12 months after a single ESI with 60 mg of methylprednisolone. One reported case of death was caused by complications after epidural hematoma. Of the permanent spinal cord injuries, 2 were caused by direct trauma, 3 were caused by epidural hematoma, and in one case there was no apparent trauma. The investigators noted that many of the severe complications could be avoided by precise needle placement and careful technique. Bleeding diathesis and thus potential for hematoma could theoretically be avoided with a careful patient history. Only one of the 3 epidural hematomas cited, however, was clearly associated with anticoagulation or antiplatelet medication.

For TF ESI, the minor complications are similar to the IL route, although major complications are more frequent. Initially, case reports related to the risk of cervical spinal cord and brain injury with cervical TF ESIs raised awareness of potential serious complications. In 2007, a large retrospective anonymous survey of the American Pain Society asked physicians to report known complications of cervical TF ESIs.[9] A total of 21.4% (287/1340) responded, reporting 74 major complications (lasting >24 hours). Many of these were purportedly due to inadvertent intrarterial injection of particulate steroid causing embolism in the brain and/or spinal cord. In 2010, a review of the literature on complications of cervical TF ESIs cited 105 published major complications, 68 of these with details available.[10] Complications included brain infarction and edema, spinal cord infarction, cortical blindness, high spinal anesthesia, seizure, and bleeding. Fifteen of these led to death. Another 35 cases of major complication are referred to in the literature, but have not been published.[10] The exact number of major complications is unknown. Some practitioners argue that anonymous surveys may overestimate the number of these cases, because more than one physician could report the same case. On the other hand, because of medical-legal issues, the number of major complications may be underestimated. The proposed mechanisms of severe spinal cord and brain injuries include injection of particulate steroid into vertebral or cervical radicular arteries, needle-induced dissection/thrombosis/vasospasm, and intraarterial injection of anesthetic or pharmaceutical preservatives/vehicles. Needle misplacement is the primary mechanism by which these occur.

ANATOMY RELEVANT TO CERVICAL ESI

Performing technically sound injections to maximize efficacy and minimize risk requires exact knowledge of the anatomy. The epidural space contains the spinal nerve roots and their dural sleeves, the internal vertebral venous plexus, loose areolar tissue, segmental blood supply, adipose tissue, and lymphatics. The location of the dura is an obvious consideration, and the vascular structures are even more important. The epidural veins form an arcuate pattern, positioned laterally at the level of each vertebral body. This consideration is important for IL ESIs because venous puncture is more likely to occur laterally than with midline approaches.[11] Venous injection may not typically cause serious injury, but it decreases or voids the efficacy of the injection because the medications are dispersed into the circulation.

Key anatomic features of the cervical spine include a thin ligamentum flavum (unfused in the midline in approximately half of individuals), absence of the interspinous ligament, and a small posterior epidural space (distance between the ligamentum flavum and dura mater).[11,12] At C6 to 7 and C7 to T1, where the epidural space is the widest and most IL ESIs are placed, the mean width is 3 mm (1–4 mm).[13]

The cervical arterial anatomy within and near the intervertebral foramina is pertinent to TF ESIs. The vertebral artery is an obvious hazard. Although it typically lies anterior in the foramen, some individuals may have a tortuous vertebral artery with a more posterior location near the target for injection in the posterior foramen. Also vulnerable are spinal branches of the ascending and deep cervical arteries contributing to radicular or segmental medullary branches to the anterior spinal artery supplying the anterior spinal cord. Injury or injection of embolizing matter to these spinal branches can cause anterior spinal cord injury (**Fig. 1**).[14] In addition, these branches anastomose with branches from the vertebral artery and could jeopardize brainstem and cerebellar tissues supplied by the vertebral circulation. These spinal arterial branches can enter the foramen posteriorly, at the usual location for TF ESI needle placement.[14] Therefore, appropriate technique with consideration and knowledge of the anatomy and its appearance on fluoroscopic images is critical to avoid serious complications.

ESI APPROACHES, EVIDENCE, AND EFFICACY

Techniques available to access the cervical epidural space include the IL and TF approach. The TF route has become more common because it may place the medication more directly at the site of the proposed cause of pain. Prospective studies by Derby and others in the 1990s described improved outcomes using the TF route for radicular pain in the lumbar spine.[15,16] Similar studies comparing the IL and TF routes are not available for the cervical spine, although there is some evidence to suggest the TF route has advantages for certain diagnoses. The varied ESI techniques and diversity of etiologies of radicular pain make the comparison of studies difficult, and it is likely that all types of ESIs are not equally efficacious for all causes of radiculopathy.

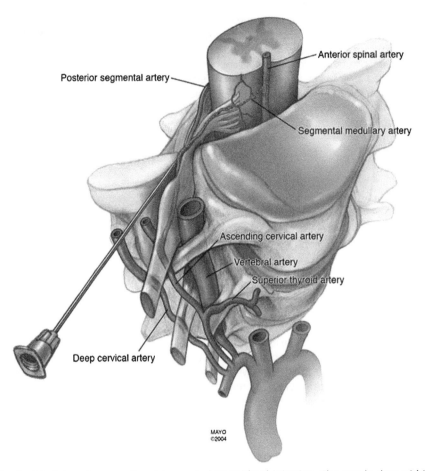

Fig. 1. Arterial anatomy pertinent to cervical TF epidural injection. The purple dots within the anterior spinal artery symbolize where intraarterial particulate matter could terminate and embolize. (By permission of Mayo Foundation for Medical Education and Research. All rights reserved.)

The next sections provide an overview of the literature and are not intended to serve as a reference for conducting the procedures.

Fluoroscopy

The use of fluoroscopic guidance for epidural needle placement in the cervical spine is considered standard of care. Fluoroscopy is used in conjunction with radiopaque contrast to establish correct epidural placement without intravascular injection. In the past, IL placement was sometimes made without fluoroscopic guidance. However, inaccurate needle placement occurs in 17% to 53% of IL injections performed without fluoroscopic guidance.[17–21]

For TF ESI, fluoroscopy is mandatory along with the use of real-time fluoroscopy or digital subtraction angiography to assess for vascular injection. Negative aspiration is not a reliable means of detecting intravascular placement. Greater than 50% of cases in which intravascular placement was documented by digital subtraction angiography had negative aspiration.[22] The documentation of epidural flow also does not rule out vascular injection, because a combination of epidural and vascular flow is often encountered. Real-time or live fluoroscopy is performed by continuous fluoroscopy while contrast media is injected. Digital subtraction angiography is performed in the same manner by the physician, but requires additional software that "subtracts" stationary objects on the fluoroscopic image and shows only moving or new objects. With this software, vascular structures are not obscured by radiopaque structures and are more readily visualized. Digital subtraction angiography has been shown to be superior to live fluoroscopy in the cervical spine in which the rate of detection of intravascular injection nearly doubled to 32.8% compared with 17.9% with real-time fluoroscopy.[23]

Injectate

There are no standardized practices for the type and volume of medication administered via an epidural injection, and there is significant variation across disciplines and institutions. A steroid/local anesthetic mixture is the most commonly used for ESI in both academic institutions and private practices.[24] The volume of the injectate varies based on the approach used. Generally, volumes do not exceed 2 to 3 mL for TF and 3 to 4 mL for cervical IL ESIs.[25] Some argue that larger volumes may dilute the injectate and lessen effects at a specific target.

More recently, the question of risks and efficacy of particulate versus nonparticulate steroids for TF ESIs has been raised. Given the risk of intraarterial injection and neurologic sequelae described earlier, most physicians now use nonparticulate steroid for cervical TF ESIs. Intraarterial injection of nonparticulate steroid did not cause embolic injury in one animal study. In this study, direct injection of steroid into the vertebral artery of pigs showed none that received particulate steroid (methylprednisolone) regained consciousness, whereas all of those that were administered nonparticulate steroid showed no evidence of neurologic injury and no changes were noted on magnetic resonance imaging.[26] Therefore, if inadvertent intraarterial injection were to occur during TF ESI, nonparticulate steroid should not result in neurologic injury.

However, there is some debate that particulate steroids may not be as efficacious as nonparticulate steroids. In 2006, a small study comparing effectiveness in cervical TF ESI noted that there was no statistically significant difference, but there was a trend favoring particulate steroids.[27] In 2009, a larger retrospective study comparing triamcinolone (particulate) versus dexamethasone (nonparticulate) in cervical TF ESI for cervical radiculopathy found no significant difference in effectiveness or in the rate of those who went on to have surgery.[28] However, there is a lumbar TF study that suggests pain scores are significantly more improved with triamcinolone versus dexamethasone at 1 month.[29] Limitations of this study include that the baseline pain scores were significantly different between groups, confounding the results. In addition, there was not a significant difference in Oswestry disability scores between groups. Overall, nonparticulate steroid is nearly or equally effective as particulate steroids in cervical TF ESI for the treatment of radiculopathy and carries less risk of causing major neurologic injury.

IL Approach

Technique

The IL technique achieves access to the epidural space using a midline approach preferably one spinal segment below the suspected disease site because most epidural spread is cephlad. The route of the needle from superficial to deep includes the skin, subcutaneous tissue, nuchal ligament, ligamentum flavum (although it is thin and often absent in the midline), then entry into the epidural space. Physicians avoid the IL approach if there has been surgery at the site of intended injection, especially laminectomy, given derangement of the anatomy and a higher risk of dural puncture. The most common technique includes a loss of resistance technique used to identify entry into the epidural space, which can be lost with epidural scarring. Fluoroscopy with radiopaque contrast confirms epidural placement and excludes vascular flow. Medication is then injected and postinjection washout images are taken to confirm flow of the medication to the target.

Evidence

Several retrospective and one prospective controlled study have been conducted on cervical IL ESIs for neck pain and radiculopathy performed without fluoroscopy.[30,31] Success for the treatment of radiculopathy was cited at 40% to 60%. However, the rate of misplacement of a cervical IL ESI without fluoroscopic guidance has been cited as high as 53%,[21] and these results, therefore, are difficult to interpret.

Studies on cervical IL ESIs with fluoroscopic guidance have also provided favorable evidence, although none of these are randomized controlled studies. In a prospective study of 13 patients with cervical disc herniation with neck pain and radiculopathy who had up to 3 cervical ESIs (proceeding from blind IL to fluoroscopically guided IL to fluoroscopically guided TF) all patients had resolution of symptoms at 12-month follow-up, except for one with neck pain.[32] A retrospective study of 91 patients with neck pain and radiculopathy showed 72% achieved success, but follow-up was only 2 weeks.[33] A study of physical therapy (and other noninterventional care) combined with cervical IL ESI with fluoroscopic guidance (only for persistent symptoms after noninterventional care) showed that 20 of 26 patients with cervical radiculopathy and disc herniation had good to excellent results.[34] Most of these patients had neurologic deficits, yet were able to avoid surgery.

Studies have also aimed to identify which causes of cervical radiculopathy respond best to IL ESI. Kwon and colleagues[33] showed that patients with osseous central and foraminal stenosis had less improvement than those with a disc herniation. In 2009, a retrospective study of 32 patients with cervical radiculopathy treated with fluoroscopically guided IL ESI with a catheter guided to the level of symptoms found that the presence of central canal stenosis correlated with significantly better outcome as measured by change in Neck Disability Index.[35] Overall, it is unclear if a specific cause of cervical radiculopathy is more responsive to IL ESI.

TF Approach

Technique

The TF approach is considered to be more specific, delivering the injectate directly to the site of disease at the ventral epidural space next to the disc, the dorsal root ganglion, and the nerve root. The technique involves using fluoroscopy to identify a subpedicular target within the intervertebral foramen.

The correct oblique view of the target foramen is obtained with fluoroscopy. An entry point overlying the posterior half of the target foramen is used to pass a needle into the neck. Care is taken to ensure that the tip of the needle is positioned over the anterior half of the superior articular process to ensure that it is not inserted too far into the foramen. The needle is advanced to the superior articular process and then readjusted to enter the foramen tangential to its posterior wall, opposite the equator of the foramen. Accurate placement is confirmed in multiple planes with radiopaque contrast and fluoroscopy.[36]

Real-time or live fluoroscopy or digital subtraction angiography is used to rule out vascular flow. The anesthetic is injected first, and a pause of 60 to 90 seconds is conducted to monitor for side effects in the central nervous system, which may be reversible (seizures, transient paresis, and respiratory depression), as an additional indicator of anesthetic intravascular injection. The medication is then injected and postinjection washout images are taken to confirm flow of the medication to the target.

Selective nerve root block

In practice and in the literature, the terms selective nerve root block (SNRB) and TF ESI are sometimes used interchangeably. The term SNRB describes a highly selective TF injection in which the interventionalist anesthetizes a single specific nerve root to confirm or refute it as the source of pain.[37] The selective nature of the nerve root block applies if the injectate/anesthetic travels only to the target nerve root. However, it has recently been shown that with as little as 0.5 mL of contrast directed via SNRB at L4 or L5, flow to an adjacent level can be seen.[38] With standard doses of 1 to 2 mL of anesthetic used, these injections are likely often nonselective or at least only partially selective.

Evidence

For lumbar radicular pain, 2 recent randomized controlled trials support the efficacy of TF ESI, with decreased surgical rates and decreased pain scores at 12-month follow-up.[39,40] There are no randomized controlled studies to show efficacy of TF ESIs in the cervical spine. However, several case series show favorable results.[32,41–44] Results tended to be better in those more than 50 years old[42] and in patients with nontraumatic radiculopathy.[43,45,46] To determine effect on surgery sparing, a small series of 21 patients with cervical radiculopathy awaiting surgery underwent 2 TF ESIs 2 weeks apart.[47] Five of the 21 patients had excellent results at 4 months and elected not to have surgery. However, there was no control group to show if this was a better outcome than natural history alone. A recent prospective randomized trial of 40 patients with cervical radiculopathy resulting from degenerative changes, all with positive response to SNRB, did not show an increased benefit of methylprednisolone over bupivicaine alone at 3-week follow-up.[48] Limitations of this study include that the questionnaire used was not a validated outcome measure and inclusion criteria required only 50% relief of extremity pain with the SNRB. In addition, these findings may be limited to TF ESIs for cervical radiculopathy due to degenerative causes, and better results with corticosteroids would be expected for soft disc herniations in which inflammation may play a larger role.

IL Versus TF

Injectate flow

The rationale for using a TF approach in preference to the IL approach is that it delivers the medication directly to the ventral epidural space, closer to the target disc and/or nerve root. Studies evaluating contrast patterns generally support this concept in the lumbar spine. Though, a recent analysis of contrast patterns for midline cervical IL ESIs found the rate of ventral epidural spread was 56.7% with 1 mL and 90% with 2 mL of injectate.[49]

Evidence

Studies of lumbar TF ESIs demonstrate benefit over IL approach in the lumbar spine.[50] Comparison studies have not been conducted in the cervical spine, although some extrapolation may be reasonable. In a study of 48 patients with cervical radiculopathy who did not improve with IL ESI, 79.2% were reported to have an effective TF ESI.[28]

In these patients who had failed IL ESI, patients with foraminal stenosis were more likely to improve than those with disc herniation. TF ESIs have a theoretic benefit over IL ESIs, and may be superior for certain causes of radiculopathy, but this has not been clearly substantiated in the cervical spine. Given the increased risk of major complications with TF ESI discussed earlier, the potential benefit must be carefully weighed for each individual patient.

ESI CONCLUSIONS

Neither TF nor IL ESIs have been studied against a control for the treatment of cervical radicular pain. Retrospective and prospective series overall do suggest favorable results for short-term improvement. Patients with radiculopathy and central stenosis have been shown to have better outcomes after cervical IL ESI, but radiculopathy with disc herniation has also been shown to have better outcomes than osseous central or foraminal stenosis. For cervical TF ESIs, patients with nontraumatic cervical radiculopathy and patients more than 50 years old tend to do better. However, one study for cervical radiculopathy resulting from degenerative changes has shown that the addition of corticosteroid to bupivicaine alone does not have added benefit.[48] Without clear evidence of which patients respond best to cervical ESI, is it up to the physician to make a well-informed and conscientious decision for each case.

There is greater risk of major and devastating complications with cervical TF ESI compared with IL ESI related to the risk of arterial puncture and injection. The use of fluoroscopy, especially in combination with digital subtraction angiography, minimizes this risk, and the use of nonparticulate steroid may obviate this risk. Given the clearly better safety profile of nonparticulate steroids and the paucity of data supporting the superiority of particulate over nonparticulate steroid, cervical TF ESI should be performed with nonparticulate steroid until studies prove otherwise.

Well-executed noninterventional care can also provide favorable outcomes, and should be initiated before ESI. In one study of noninterventional care combined with IL ESI if needed, 92.3% of patients with cervical radiculopathy and disc herniation avoided surgery.[34] Only 35% of these patients received a single IL ESI. Cervical ESIs should not be a first-line treatment of cervical radiculopathy and should be considered only in conjunction with a rational and comprehensive rehabilitation treatment plan.

REFERENCES

1. Lievre JA, Bloch-Michel H, Attali P. [Epidural hydrocortisone in the treatment of sciatica]. Rev Rhum Mal Osteoartic 1955;22(9–10):696–7 [in French].
2. Thierry-Mieg J. [Cervical epidural injections of corticoids in hyperalgic cervico-brachial neuralgias. 1st cervical epidurographical pictures]. Rev Rhum Mal Osteoartic 1961;28: 451–3 [in French].
3. Benzon HT. Epidural steroid injections for low back pain and lumbosacral radiculopathy. Pain 1986;24(3):277–95.
4. Gardner WJ, Goebert HW Jr, Sehgal AD. Intraspinal corticosteroids in the treatment of sciatica. Trans Am Neurol Assoc 1961;86:214–5.
5. Saal JS, Franson RC, Dobrow R, et al. High levels of inflammatory phospholipase A2 activity in lumbar disc herniations. Spine (Phila Pa 1976) 1990;15(7):674–8.
6. Furusawa N, Baba H, Miyoshi N, et al. Herniation of cervical intervertebral disc: immunohistochemical examination and measurement of nitric oxide production. Spine (Phila Pa 1976) 2001;26(10):1110–6.

7. Kang JD, Georgescu HI, McIntyre-Larkin L, et al. Herniated cervical intervertebral discs spontaneously produce matrix metalloproteinases, nitric oxide, interleukin-6, and prostaglandin E2. Spine (Phila Pa 1976) 1995;20(22):2373–8.
8. Abbasi A, Malhotra G, Malanga G, et al. Complications of interlaminar cervical epidural steroid injections: a review of the literature. Spine (Phila Pa 1976) 2007;32(19):2144–51.
9. Scanlon GC, Moeller-Bertram T, Romanowsky SM, et al. Cervical transforaminal epidural steroid injections: more dangerous than we think? Spine (Phila Pa 1976) 2007;32(11):1249–56.
10. Benny B, Azari P, Briones D. Complications of cervical transforaminal epidural steroid injections. Am J Phys Med Rehabil 2010;89(7):601–17.
11. Raj P, editor. Pain medicine a comprehensive review. St Louis (MO): Mosby; 1996.
12. Hogan QH. Epidural anatomy examined by cryomicrotome section. Influence of age, vertebral level, and disease. Reg Anesth 1996;21(5):395–406.
13. Aldrete JA, Mushin AU, Zapata JC, et al. Skin to cervical epidural space distances as read from magnetic resonance imaging films: consideration of the "hump pad". J Clin Anesth 1998;10(4):309–13.
14. Huntoon MA. Anatomy of the cervical intervertebral foramina: vulnerable arteries and ischemic neurologic injuries after transforaminal epidural injections. Pain 2005;117(1–2):104–11.
15. Derby R, Kine G, Saal JA, et al. Response to steroid and duration of radicular pain as predictors of surgical outcome. Spine (Phila Pa 1976) 1992;17(Suppl 6): S176–83.
16. Lutz GE, Vad VB, Wisneski RJ. Fluoroscopic transforaminal lumbar epidural steroids: an outcome study. Arch Phys Med Rehabil 1998;79(11):1362–6.
17. Renfrew DL, Moore TE, Kathol MH, et al. Correct placement of epidural steroid injections: fluoroscopic guidance and contrast administration. AJNR Am J Neuroradiol 1991;12(5):1003–7.
18. Stitz MY, Sommer HM. Accuracy of blind versus fluoroscopically guided caudal epidural injection. Spine (Phila Pa 1976) 1999;24(13):1371–6.
19. White AH, Derby R, Wynne G. Epidural injections for the diagnosis and treatment of low-back pain. Spine (Phila Pa 1976) 1980;5(1):78–86.
20. Mehta M, Salmon N. Extradural block. Confirmation of the injection site by X-ray monitoring. Anaesthesia 1985;40(10):1009–12.
21. Stojanovic MP, Vu TN, Caneris O, et al. The role of fluoroscopy in cervical epidural steroid injections: an analysis of contrast dispersal patterns. Spine (Phila Pa 1976) 2002;27(5):509–14.
22. Furman MB, Giovanniello MT, O'Brien EM. Incidence of intravascular penetration in transforaminal cervical epidural steroid injections. Spine (Phila Pa 1976) 2003; 28(1):21–5.
23. McLean JP, Sigler JD, Plastaras CT, et al. The rate of detection of intravascular injection in cervical transforaminal epidural steroid injections with and without digital subtraction angiography. PM R 2009;1(7):636–42.
24. Cluff R, Mehio AK, Cohen SP, et al. The technical aspects of epidural steroid injections: a national survey. Anesth Analg 2002;95(2):403–8.
25. Chen B, Stitik TP. Epidural steroid injections. Emedicine 2009. Available at: http://emedicine.medscape.com/article/325733-overview. Accessed October 25, 2010.
26. Okubadejo GO, Talcott MR, Schmidt RE, et al. Perils of intravascular methylprednisolone injection into the vertebral artery. An animal study. J Bone Joint Surg Am 2008;90(9):1932–8.

27. Dreyfuss P, Baker R, Bogduk N. Comparative effectiveness of cervical transforaminal injections with particulate and nonparticulate corticosteroid preparations for cervical radicular pain. Pain Med 2006;7(3):237–42.
28. Lee JW, Park KW, Chung SK, et al. Cervical transforaminal epidural steroid injection for the management of cervical radiculopathy: a comparative study of particulate versus non-particulate steroids. Skeletal Radiol 2009;38(11):1077–82.
29. Park CH, Lee SH, Kim BI. Comparison of the effectiveness of lumbar transforaminal epidural injection with particulate and nonparticulate corticosteroids in lumbar radiating pain. Pain Med 2010;11(11):1654–8.
30. Ferrante FM, Wilson SP, Iacobo C, et al. Clinical classification as a predictor of therapeutic outcome after cervical epidural steroid injection. Spine (Phila Pa 1976) 1993;18(6):730–6.
31. Stav A, Ovadia L, Sternberg A, et al. Cervical epidural steroid injection for cervicobrachialgia. Acta Anaesthesiol Scand 1993;37(6):562–6.
32. Bush K, Hillier S. Outcome of cervical radiculopathy treated with periradicular/epidural corticosteroid injections: a prospective study with independent clinical review. Eur Spine J 1996;5(5):319–25.
33. Kwon JW, Lee JW, Kim SH, et al. Cervical interlaminar epidural steroid injection for neck pain and cervical radiculopathy: effect and prognostic factors. Skeletal Radiol 2007;36(5):431–6.
34. Saal JS, Saal JA, Yurth EF. Nonoperative management of herniated cervical intervertebral disc with radiculopathy. Spine (Phila Pa 1976) 1996;21(16):1877–83.
35. Fish DE, Kobayashi HW, Chang TL, et al. MRI prediction of therapeutic response to epidural steroid injection in patients with cervical radiculopathy. Am J Phys Med Rehabil 2009;88(3):239–46.
36. Rathmell JP, Aprill C, Bogduk N. Cervical transforaminal injection of steroids. Anesthesiology 2004;100(6):1595–600.
37. Furman MB, Lee TS, Mehta A, et al. Contrast flow selectivity during transforaminal lumbosacral epidural steroid injections. Pain Physician 2008;11(6):855–61.
38. Vassiliev D. Spread of contrast during L4 and L5 nerve root infiltration under fluoroscopic guidance. Pain Physician 2007;10(3):461–6.
39. Riew KD, Yin Y, Gilula L, et al. The effect of nerve-root injections on the need for operative treatment of lumbar radicular pain. A prospective, randomized, controlled, double-blind study. J Bone Joint Surg Am 2000;82-A(11):1589–93.
40. Vad VB, Bhat AL, Lutz GE, et al. Transforaminal epidural steroid injections in lumbosacral radiculopathy: a prospective randomized study. Spine (Phila Pa 1976) 2002;27(1):11–6.
41. Vallee JN, Feydy A, Carlier RY, et al. Chronic cervical radiculopathy: lateral-approach periradicular corticosteroid injection. Radiology 2001;218(3):886–92.
42. Lin EL, Lieu V, Halevi L, et al. Cervical epidural steroid injections for symptomatic disc herniations. J Spinal Disord Tech 2006;19(3):183–6.
43. Slipman CW, Lipetz JS, Jackson HB, et al. Therapeutic selective nerve root block in the nonsurgical treatment of atraumatic cervical spondylotic radicular pain: a retrospective analysis with independent clinical review. Arch Phys Med Rehabil 2000;81(6):741–6.
44. Cyteval C, Thomas E, Decoux E, et al. Cervical radiculopathy: open study on percutaneous periradicular foraminal steroid infiltration performed under CT control in 30 patients. AJNR Am J Neuroradiol 2004;25(3):441–5.
45. Slipman CW, Lipetz JS, DePalma MJ, et al. Therapeutic selective nerve root block in the nonsurgical treatment of traumatically induced cervical spondylotic radicular pain. Am J Phys Med Rehabil 2004;83(6):446–54.

46. Slipman CW, Lipetz JS, Jackson HB, et al. Outcomes of therapeutic selective nerve root blocks for whiplash induced cervical radicular pain. Pain Physician 2001;4(2):167–74.
47. Kolstad F, Leivseth G, Nygaard OP. Transforaminal steroid injections in the treatment of cervical radiculopathy. A prospective outcome study. Acta Neurochir (Wien) 2005;147(10):1065–70 [discussion: 1070].
48. Anderberg L, Annertz M, Persson L, et al. Transforaminal steroid injections for the treatment of cervical radiculopathy: a prospective and randomised study. Eur Spine J 2007;16(3):321–8.
49. Kim KS, Shin SS, Kim TS, et al. Fluoroscopically guided cervical interlaminar epidural injections using the midline approach: an analysis of epidurography contrast patterns. Anesth Analg 2009;108(5):1658–61.
50. Schaufele MK, Hatch L, Jones W. Interlaminar versus transforaminal epidural injections for the treatment of symptomatic lumbar intervertebral disc herniations. Pain Physician 2006;9(4):361–6.

Surgical Treatment and Outcomes of Lumbar Radiculopathy

Adam J. Bruggeman, MD, Robert C. Decker, MD*

KEYWORDS

- Radiculopathy • Treatment outcome
- Lumbar vertebrae/surgery • Diskectomy
- Sciatica • Cauda equina

The first discussion of operative management for lumbar radiculopathy due to a herniated disk was introduced by Mixter and Barr in 1934.[1] In this report of 19 cases using a complete laminectomy and transdural approach, they began a debate that has continued over 75 years. Shortly after that landmark paper, Love[2] and Semmes[3] described the extradural, hemilaminectomy approach for removal of an intervertebral disk herniation. In 1964, Smith[4] reported on a new substance, chymopapain, which could dissolve the nucleus pulposus and provide a less invasive way to manage a herniated disk. He reported on 10 human and 22 canine cases with good results. Caspar,[5] Yasargil,[6] and Williams[7] subsequently described the first microsurgical approaches to the lumbar spine. The enthusiasm for minimally invasive surgery continued with Forst and Hausmann[8] describing the use of an arthroscope for visualization of the intervertebral disk. This was followed by Foley and colleagues[9] nearly 15 years later, who described a microendoscopic technique for lumbar decompression.

Today's surgeons use many of these techniques to treat lumbar disk herniations, which are a common cause of radiculopathy. The incidence of sciatica reported in the literature varies from 5%[10] to 14%.[11] Several studies have estimated the costs of low back pain as a whole, of which lumbar disk disease encompasses a portion of these costs ranging from $84 billion to $624 billion in the United States.[12]

With the current health care climate and economic situation, great attention has been paid to best practices in lumbar spine surgery in the medical and popular literature. Weber[13] published his often-quoted study on the natural history of lumbar disk herniation in 1982, concluding that surgical intervention has improved outcomes over nonsurgical management, at least in the short term. The Maine study was the first large-scale randomized trial, and the investigators provided results at the 1-year,[14]

Disclosures: Dr Bruggeman owns stock in and has an immediate family member who is an employee of Exactech, Incorporated (Gainesville, FL).
Department of Orthopaedics and Rehabilitation, University of Florida, 3450 Hull Road, Gainesville, FL 32607, USA
* Corresponding author.
E-mail address: deckerc@ortho.ufl.edu

Phys Med Rehabil Clin N Am 22 (2011) 161–177
doi:10.1016/j.pmr.2010.10.002
1047-9651/11/$ – see front matter © 2011 Elsevier Inc. All rights reserved.

5-year,[15] and 10-year[16] intervals. More recently, the 2- and 4-year outcomes from the multi-center Spine Patient Outcomes Research Trial (SPORT) were published.[17,18] The results of the SPORT trial have graced the front pages of newspapers and magazines, and it has generated significant discussion among practitioners and nonpractitioners alike.

PATHOPHYSIOLOGY OF RADICULOPATHY

To justify surgery for radiculopathy, one must prove that surgery actually relieves the cause of the radiculopathy. Although the causes of radiculopathy are not fully understood, Olmarker and colleagues performed a series of studies on pigs that provide some answers. It is useful to divide those causes of radiculopathy into 2 main categories: mechanical and chemical.

Mechanical

Spinal nerve roots, although well protected by the vertebral column from outside compression, are particularly susceptible to compression from objects that arise from within the vertebral column. They lack the perineurium and epineurium that are seen in peripheral nerves. Their vascular supply is also more easily compromised.[19] Two studies were done before Olmarker's series of studies that showed that spinal nerve roots were more susceptible to compression than peripheral nerve roots.[20,21] Olmarker and colleagues[22] showed over several publications that spinal nerve roots, when compressed, exhibited intraneural edema, deprived nutritional supply,[23] and loss of amplitude of nerve conduction.[24] The nerve conduction study also demonstrated that more rapid compression and higher pressures have a deleterious effect on recovery of nerve function. These findings were confirmed in awake surgical patients. In the study by Kuslich and colleagues,[25] noncompressed nerve roots did not reproduce the patient's pain when stimulated intraoperatively. However, stimulation of compressed nerve roots consistently reproduced the patient's preoperative symptoms.

Chemical

Olmarker followed his mechanical studies on porcine cauda equina with further studies on the effects of autologous nucleus pulposus on spinal nerve roots. His group first showed that autologous nucleus pulposus applied to nerve roots without mechanical compression caused statistically significant changes in nerve conduction velocity when compared with nerve roots that had epidural fat applied to them.[26] Electron microscopic examination of the nerves revealed that the changes were not limited to nerve conduction but also caused axonal injury and Schwann-cell damage.[27] Follow-up studies demonstrated inflammatory changes induced by the nucleus pulposus, including leukotaxis and increased vascular permeability.[28] This inflammation was then attributed in part to tumor necrosis factor α.[29] Inhibition of this substance reversed the effects in pig models,[30] but human studies have failed to show effectiveness of treatment with antibody to tumor necrosis factor α.[31,32]

NATURAL HISTORY OF THE HERNIATED LUMBAR DISK

To fully understand the benefits of surgery, the natural history of *untreated* lumbar disk herniations must be established as a benchmark. Bozzao and colleagues[33] demonstrated a reduction in size of disk herniation of at least 30% in 63% of patients. Clinical symptoms worsened in only 8% in that study. Saal and Saal[34] performed a retrospective cohort study on 64 patients, and their patient series had 90%

good-to-excellent outcomes and 92% return-to-work status. Both studies suffer from small sample sizes and difficulty in maintaining patients in the nonoperative group.

Three major randomized trials have investigated surgical and nonsurgical management of the herniated lumbar disk. The nonoperative groups in each of these studies are also important for providing information on the outcomes of nonoperative management. One major difficulty in combining this information is the heterogeneous nature of the nonoperative options presented to patients and used in these studies.

Weber's research in 1982 reported on a group of 66 patients (of 126) who were randomized to nonoperative management. Forty-nine of those 66 patients remained in the nonoperative arm. Within that group, the patients reported 55% good outcomes, and 76% were without pain at 10 years. Shorter term outcomes were less promising, with a similar number reporting good outcomes, but only 53% reporting no pain at 4 years.[13]

The Maine Lumbar Spine Study provided results at varying intervals for a group of 170 patients. The early results showed that leg pain was improved in 56% of patients at 1 year,[14] 60% at 5 years,[15] and 64% at 10 years.[16] Patient satisfaction was reported as 40% at 1 year,[14] 46% at 5 years,[15] and 56% at 10 years.[16] The results follow a similar trend to Weber's results, with gradual improvement over several years and just over half the respondents satisfied with their outcomes.

The most recent multi-center trial, SPORT, encompassed a randomized group and an observational cohort. The high crossover rates in this study lead to difficulty interpreting the data; therefore, this article focuses on the observational cohort group of 191 subjects in the nonoperative group. Pain scores were measured with the Short Form-36 (SF-36) Bodily Pain scale. These scores improved 26.0 points at 3 months, 32.0 points at 1 year, and 32.4 points at 2 years.[17] When combining the observational and randomized nonoperative groups, SF-36 scores improved 30.7 points at 4 years.[18] Patients reported satisfaction with their treatment at a rate of 29.4% at 3 months, 44.7% at 1 year, and 49.1% at 2 years.[17] When combining the 2 nonoperative groups over time, the overall satisfaction rate without surgery was 61.3%.[18]

SURGICAL OPTIONS

Since 1939, many approaches to lumbar diskectomy have been described (**Fig. 1**). Three techniques encompass most of the surgical approaches used in practice today. Each has advantages and disadvantages, and studies have been done over the last decade to compare the outcomes and complications of these techniques.

Open Diskectomy Technique

Although Mixter and Barr[1] described the first open approach in 1934, this approach required a complete laminectomy and was transdural. Love[2] and Semmes[3] modified this approach by performing a hemilaminectomy with an extradural approach.

The patient is placed prone on a radiolucent table and the lumbar spine is flexed to open the interlaminar space. Using a spinal needle and intraoperative fluoroscopy, the correct level is identified. Incision is made in the midline, centered over the spinous processes, and is approximately 4 to 6 cm long. The incision can be performed as far proximally and distally as is required to remove disk material and obtain good visualization. Dissection is continued through the fat and fascia down to the spinous processes. Using a Cobb elevator and electrocautery, the multifidus (and longissimus as necessary) is dissected subperiosteally on the affected side, exposing the lamina and facet joint as dissection continues laterally. Retractors are placed to hold the paraspinal muscles out of the operative field. The ligamentum flavum is identified in the

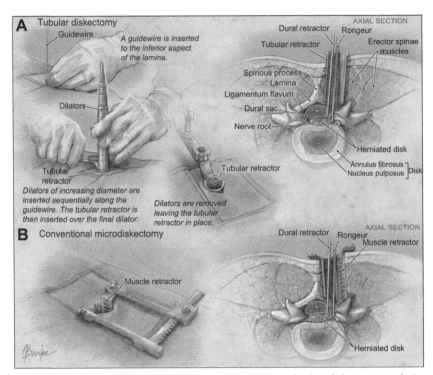

Fig. 1. Comparison of tubular diskectomy and conventional microdiskectomy techniques (A–B). (From Arts MP, Brand R, van den Akker ME, et al. Tubular diskectomy vs conventional microdiskectomy for sciatica: a randomized controlled trial. JAMA 2009;302:151. Copyright © 2009 American Medical Association. All rights reserved.)

interlaminar space and sharply incised. Using Kerrison rongeur, the ligamentum flavum and hemilamina are removed at the level of the pathology. Alternatively, the bone removal can be done with a high-speed burr. In the depth of the incision, the dural sac is identified and carefully dissected off the floor of the spinal canal. The dural sac and nerve root are retracted medially with a right-angled nerve retractor to expose the intervertebral disk. The posterior longitudinal ligament is incised with a long-handled blade, and herniated disk material is removed.

Conventional Microdiskectomy

Yasargil[6] and Caspar[5] published articles outlining the microdiskectomy approach in 1977. Shortly thereafter, Williams[7] published his series of patients, many of whom were Las Vegas showgirls in search of a more cosmetic procedure for lumbar disk disease. His satisfactory results in 91% of patients helped to popularize the procedure.

This procedure was originally described for a patient to be placed in the lateral decubitus position with the affected side up but is also performed with the patient in the prone position as previously described. In this approach, the skin incision is made just lateral to the spinous process instead of directly over the spinous processes, as in the open procedure. Incision is typically only 2 cm long for a single-level diskectomy. The fascia is incised just a few millimeters lateral to the spinous process, and dissection is then carried subperiosteally to identify the inferior third of the superior lamina at the 12 o'clock position, the medial aspect of the facet joint laterally, and the superior third of the inferior lamina at the 6 o'clock position, with the interlaminar space and ligamentum flavum in the center of the field. The operative microscope is typically used to develop the surgical interval through this small incision, and various retractors have been developed along with coaxial lighting to assist with visualization. Depending on the positioning of the patient and the level of surgery, a portion of the lamina and facet are removed with high-speed burr or Kerrison rongeur. Numerous studies[35–37] have shown that up to 50% of the facet joint can be removed without destabilizing the spine. The ligamentum flavum is carefully released from the superior aspect of the inferior lamina and removed with Kerrison rongeurs, as needed, to expose the compressed nerve root. As is the case with standard open diskectomy, a right-angled nerve retractor is used to protect the dural sac and nerve root, and the posterior longitudinal ligament is incised sharply with a blade. Disk material is then removed in the standard manner.

Microendoscopic Diskectomy/Tubular Diskectomy

Foley and colleagues[9] described the endoscopic technique for microdiskectomy in 1997. They used a muscle-splitting approach as opposed to the previously described subperiosteal dissection to further reduce the trauma to the paraspinal musculature and improve results. Arthroscopic techniques are increasingly desired by patients for other orthopedic procedures, and it was only a matter of time before this was applied to the spine. Specialized instruments were required, and as these were fine-tuned, results and technical barriers improved. Those instruments and retractors have also been used for standard microdiskectomy.

For this procedure, although positioning is the same, the incision is typically made 1.5 cm lateral to the spinous process on the side of the disk herniation. The incision length is also around 1.5 cm long, depending on the size of the tubular retractors. A k-wire is inserted into the medial facet, and a series of increasingly larger diameter dilators are placed over the k-wire. The final endoscopic tube is placed around the largest dilator and secured to the bed with a flexible arm. Fluoroscopy confirms the final positioning of the tube and the inner dilators are removed. An endoscope is placed into the working portal, with other retractors and tools capable of being placed through the same portal to perform the dissection and diskectomy. The dissection and diskectomy are performed in the same fashion as described in the microdiskectomy section. Many of today's surgeons use the dilator tube as described but look down the tube with an operative microscope as opposed to an endoscope. This is sometimes referred to as tubular microdiskectomy or tubular diskectomy.

Comparison of Techniques

When multiple treatments for the same disease are developed, questions revolve around which treatment is best. Many studies have been performed to date comparing the previously mentioned surgical approaches, but the results have been mixed.

Several studies have investigated the difference between conventional open diskectomy with minimally invasive techniques. Yasargil[6] and Foley and colleagues[9] in their initial articles each reported on their techniques and on their results. They established the safety of their procedures, and subsequent articles validated the safety of the procedure and showed significant improvement in outcomes over the traditional open diskectomy.[7,38–40] These studies demonstrated a wide variety of improvements, including smaller incision, less blood loss, and quicker return to work, with similar clinical outcomes for improvement in symptoms.

Nakagawa, and colleagues,[41] published their results on 30 consecutive patients treated with Love's open method and 30 consecutive patients treated with Foley and Smith's microendoscopic method (MED). The MED group showed statistically significant improvement over the Love group for recovery rate through the first 16 weeks, creatine phosphokinase levels, and return-to-work rate (49.2 days vs 85.9 days). Recovery rate was not significantly different at 24 weeks or final follow-up. Blood loss trended toward lower and length of surgery, longer (109.1 minutes vs 79.3 minutes) with MED, but neither were significant. The increased length of surgery is potentially related to experience, because the 30 patients were very early in the investigators' adoption of the MED technique. A review of the individual cases shows a significant improvement in operative time from the first case (more than 180 minutes) to the thirtieth case (<60 minutes). Brayda-Bruno and colleagues[42] also noted the improvement in operative time with experience in their series of 68 patients, from 150 minutes to 35 minutes (average of 1 hour).

Muramatsu and colleagues[43] evaluated the microendoscopic diskectomy in a different way. His group looked at postoperative magnetic resonance imaging images of 25 patients who underwent MED and 15 who underwent standard open diskectomy (Love technique). They also reported their outcomes on 70 patients with MED procedures and 15 with open diskectomy procedures. Their results showed statistical improvement in the MED group for blood loss, analgesic requirement, number of days before ambulation, earlier return to low demand jobs, and duration of hospitalization. Radiographically, the MED group had muscular edema limited to the small incision (typically <2 cm), compared with the edema along the larger incision with the Love technique (4–5 cm). Some of the patients in the Love group demonstrated extensive edema throughout the paraspinous musculature to large areas outside of the incision area; however, no significant difference was noted in enhancement of nerve or muscle tissue between the 2 groups.

After proving the efficacy and improved morbidity of minimally invasive procedures, the 2 types of minimally invasive techniques needed to be compared and evaluated against each other. Righesso and colleagues[44] performed a prospective, randomized controlled trial on 40 patients to evaluate microdiskectomy (Caspar's technique) and MED (with an endoscope). Statistically significant improvement of the MED group over the microdiskectomy group was noted for length of hospital stay (24 hours vs 26 hours) and size of incision (2.1 cm vs 2.6 cm). The microdiskectomy group had statistically significant improvement over the MED group in operative time (63.7 minutes vs 82.6 minutes) and immediate (12 hours) postoperative pain. No statistical significance was demonstrated for blood loss, neurologic status (trend toward earlier recovery in microdiskectomy), visual analog scale (VAS) pain score after the immediate postoperative period, or Oswestry Disability Index score.

In 2008, Brock and colleagues[45] published their results on 125 patients who were prospectively randomized to a transmuscular or subperiosteal approach. This study was unable to show statistical significance for leg or back pain on the VAS, but the authors were able to show a difference favoring the transmuscular group in the postoperative Oswestry Disability Index score, as well as requirement for postoperative analgesics.

Arts and colleagues[46] performed the first double-blind randomized controlled trial in 2009 on 328 patients, comparing conventional microdiskectomy (Caspar's technique) with tubular diskectomy. The study was interesting because of its significantly larger size compared with previous studies and the double-blind randomized manner in which it was undertaken. Statistical significance was noted in favor of conventional microdiskectomy for the Roland-Morris Disability Questionnaire score at 1-year follow-up (but not earlier), operative time (36 minutes vs 47 minutes), leg pain, back pain, and general health on the VAS. The median recovery rate was 2 weeks in both groups, and rates of reherniation and blood loss were also similar. There was no significant increase in complications seen in the tubular diskectomy patients.

After a thorough review of the literature, a few recommendations can be made. Microscopic techniques seem to be superior to the traditional open technique as first described by Love. Patients tend to return to work faster, have less blood loss, and require less postoperative analgesia. Microdiskectomy, as described by Yasargil and Caspar, seems to provide similar outcomes to the more minimally invasive, transmuscular approach described by Foley and Smith. There is a significant learning curve associated with endoscopic and tubular techniques, which may provide a barrier to its incorporation into many surgeons' practice. All studies listed earlier were limited to single-level disk protrusion with sciatica, and care should be taken when applying these results to multilevel or bilateral disease.[47]

INDICATIONS FOR SURGICAL INTERVENTION

The indications for lumbar diskectomy are widely debated. Only one absolute indication for surgery exists, and that is in a patient with a documented progressive neurologic deficit. This group of patients represents a small minority of operative candidates. An ideal operative candidate is one who has failed a reasonable conservative management program and has a clinical examination that correlates with radiologic findings. Specifically, the disk herniation should be on the ipsilateral side of any neurologic deficits, and the level of pathology should be the same as the level of deficit. The definition of a reasonable conservative management program has not been clearly defined in the literature, but most studies have used 6 to 8 weeks of nonoperative management without improvement as an indication for surgery. The types of conservative management also vary widely, from physical therapy to epidural injections and everything in between. Although the surgery is typically outpatient or consists of an overnight stay, patients still require appropriate medical clearance and should be healthy enough to undergo a general anesthetic, if needed. Although these criteria represent the ideal, many patients who undergo operative treatment do not meet one or more of them.

COMPLICATIONS

All procedures carry risks, lumbar diskectomies being no different, whether they are done open or under a microscope. Dural tears are one of the more common complications,[46] particularly early in a surgeon's career. In the SPORT study,[18] dural tears were reported in 3% to 4% of cases. All their cases were done through open diskectomy. One study compared outcomes in surgeons based on their experience, finding surgeons with the least experience (50–100 prior cases) had durotomies in 7% of their cases and those in the experienced group (>500 prior cases) caused durotomy in only 0.8% of their cases.[48]

Recurrent herniation has been reviewed in many articles, highlighting its importance in terms of outcomes. The true occurrence of reherniation is unknown but varies from 5% to 15%.[18,49–51] One potential cause of reherniation is the amount of disk material removed. Limited diskectomy is removal of the extruded fragment and loose pieces of disk, typically to the posterior aspect of the vertebral wall but no further. Subtotal diskectomy is aggressive removal of nuclear material from inside the disk in addition to removal of extruded fragments and loose pieces. Carragee and colleagues[52] showed no statistical difference between subtotal and limited diskectomy, but the reherniation rate was 9% in the subtotal group and 18% in the limited group. Barth and colleagues[53] were also unable to show statistical significance between the 2 groups but did show an incidence of 10.5% in the subtotal group and 12.5% in the limited group. Although Carragee's group was unable to show a difference in reherniation rate with the amount of disk removed, an earlier study from the same group demonstrated that the size of annular defect (>6 mm in 2 planes) was associated with a much higher reoperation and multiple herniation rate.[50]

Wrong-level surgery is another cause for failure of lumbar diskectomy. Wiese and colleagues[48] noted a rate of wrong-site surgery of 1.3% in the experienced group and 3.3% in the inexperienced group, which was statistically significant. The level of surgery also seemed to change the rate of wrong site surgery. As the surgery moved further from the sacrum, the rate of wrong-level exposure increased. L5/S1 diskectomies had a rate of 0.04%, whereas L4/5 diskectomies had a rate of 4.0% and L3/4 diskectomies, 6.9%. Ammerman and colleagues[54] confirmed that level above L5/S1 has a statistically significant risk of wrong-level exposure. They also noted that advanced age (>55 years) had a higher risk of wrong-level exposure. Many have theorized that the smaller incision of a microdiskectomy or tubular diskectomy increases the risk, although this has not been proven in the literature.[46]

Wound infections are another complication seen in lumbar diskectomies. In the SPORT trial, they were reported to occur in 2% to 3% of surgeries.[18] Arts and colleagues[46] reported no wound infections in their randomized, controlled trial. Davis[55] found that wound infections were the most common complication in his group of 984 cases. The incidence of wound infections was 2.5%, with only two of the 25 infections found deep to the fascia. Wiese and colleagues[48] noted a rate of superficial infection of 1% to 2% with no cases of deep infections.

Some patients have worsening neurologic status despite surgery or due to iatrogenic causes. Nerve root injury was noted in less than 1% of patients in the SPORT study.[18] Davis noted one patient who developed paraparesis, which resolved shortly after surgery. Three patients developed paraplegia in his group.[55] Wiese noted an incidence of 0.5% to 1% worsening of neurologic status.[48]

A common dictum of spine surgeons is that diskectomy reliably improves leg pain but is not effective for, or even worsens, low back pain. Weber's original study noted that back pain occurred in 11% of patients postoperatively, although no discussion of preoperative back pain was noted.[13] In 2004, Toyone and colleagues[56] performed a prospective study on 40 patients who underwent standard diskectomy. Improvement in low back pain and leg pain was monitored according to the visual analog score. Low back pain decreased in 37 patients, had no change in one patient, slightly increased in one patient, and increased significantly in one patient. Although the back pain improvements were less dramatic than the leg pain improvements, patients with the worst back pain achieved excellent improvement, and low back pain was reliably improved with surgery. Asch and colleagues[57] found statistically significant improvements in visual analog scores for back pain in 212 consecutive patients who underwent microdiskectomy. On average, the back pain score was 7 preoperatively, improved to 3 immediately after surgery, eventually settling around 2 at final follow-up. By comparison, leg pain decreased from 7 to 0 immediately after surgery but increased to scores between 1 and 2 at final follow-up.

There are other, very rare complications, occurring in less than 1% of cases. These include injury to abdominal vascular structures or the ureter or intestinal perforation. Mortality from diskectomy is exceedingly rare but has been reported in case reports throughout the literature.

OUTCOMES TRIALS

The case for surgical management of lumbar radiculopathy secondary to lumbar disk herniation has been debated for decades. Many studies have attempted to provide clinicians with data that can assist in decision making. Despite countless hours of research and a seemingly endless number of articles in the scientific literature regarding lumbar disk herniation, there is still no clear answer on who best benefits from lumbar diskectomy. There are 2 landmark prospective studies that have significantly impacted the treatment of lumbar diskectomy.

Weber Trial

From a historical perspective, one of the first studies to discuss outcomes after randomizing patients to operative and nonoperative treatment was Weber's study from 1982.[13] He reviewed 126 patients with radiographic evidence of a lumbar disk herniation who were still symptomatic after 14 days of nonoperative management. These patients were then randomized to operative or nonoperative management. Seventeen patients in the nonoperative group crossed over into the surgical group during the first year of observation, averaging 7.5 months before surgery.

The first year's results show statistically significant improvement for the surgical group. These results were based on patient-reported satisfaction. Patients were rated as good if they stated that they were completely satisfied; fair, if satisfied with some small complaints; poor. if not satisfied and partly incapacitated; or bad, if completely incapacitated for work. Although 66% of patients achieved *good* outcomes in the surgical group, only 33% of nonoperative patients achieved good outcomes. When combining patients who achieved fair and good outcomes, 92% of the surgical group had fair or better outcomes, whereas 82% of the nonoperative group had fair or better outcomes.

At 4 and 10 years, the differences between operative and nonoperative management narrowed. The nonoperative group had 51% good outcomes, whereas the operative group remained at 70% good outcomes, excluding any patients that crossed over. At 10 years, the nonoperative group achieved 55% good outcomes and the operative group slipped to 63%. If the results of fair and good outcomes are combined, the nonoperative group achieved 90% and 92% fair or better outcomes at 4 years and 10 years, respectively. The operative group achieved 86% fair or better outcomes at 4 years and 93% at 10 years.

Weber drew several conclusions at the end of his study. The first was that the age of the patient at the time of herniation correlated with outcome at all stages of the investigation. The average age of patients that did poorly was 47 years, whereas the average age of those that did well was 40 years. At the 4-year mark, men tended to do better than women, and patients with psychosocial comorbidities tended to do worse. Many other variables did not seem to have an effect, including but not limited to occupation, neurologic examination, and level of herniation. Based on his results, Weber stated that no significant improvement was likely to occur after 4 years for either group.

Maine Lumbar Spine Study

In 1995, Atlas and colleagues[14–16] began reporting their data from a group of patients in Maine that presented with sciatica. The study was designed as a prospective cohort study, not a randomized study like Weber's. Outcomes were determined based on patient surveys that were mailed to their houses. A total of 389 patients were evaluated, with 219 treated surgically and 170, nonsurgically. The 2 groups were identical in their characteristics except that surgical patients were more often receiving worker's compensation, were more often taking narcotics, had more abnormal physical examination findings, had more severe disk disorders, and had more symptoms of sciatica overall. Open diskectomy was performed in nearly all procedures.

At 1-year follow-up, statistical significance in favor of surgical intervention was found in nearly every statistic measured. Patients improved in back and leg pain compared with baseline, SF-36 scores for physical function and bodily pain, Roland score, and satisfaction with current state. Statistical significance was not noted for worker's compensation patients. Of the surgically treated patients, 87% indicated that they would definitely or probably choose to have surgery again if they could go back in time, and 61% reported very good or excellent results. The authors also showed statistics for patients with the mildest symptoms, and, predictably, these patients did not see a significant improvement with surgical intervention when compared with nonoperative treatment.

Five-year results followed the 1-year results, with very little change in symptoms or satisfaction after 12 months. Statistical significance in favor of surgical intervention was noted for change in symptoms and functional status from baseline for low back pain, leg pain, sciatica index, and Roland Scale. Quality of life and satisfaction with current state were also significantly improved for the surgical group. Worker's compensation patients did not have statistically significant changes when they underwent surgical intervention for their sciatica. At 5 years, 63% of surgical patients (compared with 46% of the nonsurgical patients) were satisfied with their current state, and 82% of surgical patients indicated that they would still choose to have a back operation. For the least symptomatic patients, only the Roland Scale mean change showed statistical significance. Quality of life, satisfaction, sciatica frequency index, and predominant symptom improvement trended toward improvement in the surgical group, but no significance was noted.

The 10-year results were similar, but the nonoperative group showed more improvement over the last 5 years of follow-up when compared with the operative group. Statistical significance in favor of surgical improvement was still noted in change in symptoms and functional status from baseline for low back pain, leg pain, sciatica index, and modified Roland Scale. Patient satisfaction with their current state was still significant (70.5% for the surgical group and 55.5% for the nonsurgical), and 86.6% of surgical patients indicated that they would choose to undergo surgery. Worker's compensation and return to work showed no statistical improvement with surgical intervention, as was the case at 1- and 5-year follow-up.

The authors of the study noted several important trends based on their 10 years of follow-up. First, although surgical patients were significantly worse functionally and symptomatically at baseline, they were more satisfied and had better functional status at all data points. Also, surgery does not tend to affect work status or disability. Finally, patients who are reluctant to have surgery will probably have improved symptoms over time, but their improvement may not be as good as if they had chosen surgery.

SPORT Trial

The largest controlled trial to date comparing operative and nonoperative management is the SPORT trial. In this National Institute of Health-funded trial, 2 different groups were established[17,18]: one randomized and one observational. Randomized controlled trials are the gold standard for clinical trials, but experience with other similar trials in the spine literature has shown that significant crossover between operative and nonoperative groups has made interpretation of the data difficult.

An observational cohort was simultaneously studied, allowing patients to choose which treatment they would prefer from the outset. For the SPORT trial's randomized arm, 50% of the surgical group did not receive surgery, whereas 30% of the nonsurgical group did. Although there are many critiques of the SPORT trial, the investigators have produced some of the most comprehensive data available comparing operative and nonoperative management of lumbar disk herniations, with 719 patients studied in the observational cohort and 472 patients in the randomized control trial.

Following the trend of Weber's study and the Maine study, statistically significant improvement was noted at 3 months, 1 year, and 2 years in favor of surgical treatment for all primary and secondary outcomes except work status. In this study, primary outcomes were SF-36 and Oswestry Disability Index scores. Secondary outcome measures included sciatica bothersome index, work status, posttreatment satisfaction, and self-rated progress rated as major improvement. Work outcomes were worse at 6 weeks for the surgical group, equivalent at 3 and 6 months, better than nonoperative at 1 year, and equivalent again at 2 years.

Recently, the SPORT study authors released their 4-year results, with few changes from their original results. Primary outcomes showed statistically significant outcomes for the observational and randomized group when comparing the *as treated* patients (those that did not crossover) of the surgical and nonsurgical groups. The results and graphs of the *as treated* group within the randomized trial are nearly identical to those of the observational group. Secondary outcomes were also statistically significant for all measures except work status. After 4 years, the surgical group attained impressive 25-point improvements in Oswestry Disability, 31-point improvements in SF-36 bodily pain, and 30-point improvements in SF-36 physical function scores. The mean difference between the observational groups at 4 years for the Oswestry and SF-36 scores was also clinically significant, showing differences around 12 points on both scales. Finally, 77% of the surgically treated patients stated they were very or somewhat satisfied with their symptoms, whereas only 46.7% of nonoperative patients were satisfied.

OUTCOMES AND SPECIFIC GROUPS

The 3 studies discussed earlier have established that surgical treatment of sciatica due to lumbar disk herniation has some significant benefit, at least in the short term. Another question that must be answered is which populations benefit the most or least from surgical intervention. Many variables have been studied, but a few stand out in the literature and help to guide surgeons in directing their patients.

One main concern in a patient's history is the presence of a worker's compensation claim. The SPORT study was one of the only studies to show any improvement in worker's compensation patients with surgery. Their patients showed better outcomes early on, but no improvement with outcomes at 2 years.[17] Another study evaluated the development of low back pain after lumbar diskectomy, looking at the factors that lead to poor outcomes. In this study, worker's compensation patients represented 66% of the failures, and 50% of the worker's compensation patients ultimately had a failed surgery due to low back pain.[58] The Maine study demonstrated that patients with worker's compensation are as likely to continue receiving compensation regardless of whether they receive surgery.[14] Several earlier studies have shown worse outcomes with worker's compensation patients.[59–61]

The Maine study also compared patients who, at baseline, had the least symptoms. As expected, nonoperative management of patients in the lowest tertile of symptoms results in equivalent outcomes to those who have received surgery. The surgical group did show significant improvement in the Roland Scale but otherwise showed no difference in outcome.[14]

In the SPORT study, the investigators divided patients into outcomes by level of herniation. Statistical significance was seen in surgery for upper lumbar herniations (L2-3, L3-4) when compared with surgery for lower lumbar herniations (L4-5 and L5-S1). The investigators determined that patients with L2-3 and L3-4 level herniations do the best, L4-5 herniations have intermediate effects with surgery, and L5-S1 patients had the smallest treatment effects. Statistical significance was primarily seen because of worse outcomes of the nonoperative groups at the higher levels as opposed to worse surgical outcomes for the lower levels. The investigators noted that possible explanations included reduced spinal canal area at the higher lumbar levels and a higher likelihood of herniations occurring far lateral or foraminal in the higher vertebral levels.[62] Other studies have shown similar results when comparing the upper lumbar herniations to lower lumbar herniations.[63,64]

Several studies have elicited other patient characteristics that have an effect on outcome. Carragee's study in 2003 showed that annulus integrity and type of disk herniation are related to surgical outcomes. The best outcomes were seen in patients with disks that had a definitive fragment and a small tear in the annulus. Patients tended to do worse with a higher rate of reherniation and reoperation if they had the combination of extruded fragments and a large or massive annular defect or the combination of an annular bulge (no defect) with no extruded fragment. The latter group did the worst of all studied groups.[50] Another study found that poor predictors were heavy manual work, low education level, and female gender.[65]

CAUDA EQUINA SYNDROME

In the same paper that described a transdural approach to lumbar disk herniations, Mixter and Barr also provided the first description of cauda equina syndrome.[1,66] Unlike in other lumbar disk herniations in which a trial of nonoperative management is appropriate and the indications for surgery are unclear, herniations associated with cauda equina syndrome are surgical urgencies.

Signs and Symptoms

Cauda equina syndrome is classically described as the combination of saddle anesthesia, decreased or absent reflexes in the lower extremities, and neurogenic bowel or bladder dysfunction. The neurogenic bladder symptoms can reflect urinary retention or incontinence. Other associated symptoms typically include back pain and leg pain. A recent study found that the most sensitive symptoms are more than 500 mL of urinary retention in combination with 2 of the following: bilateral sciatica, subjective urinary retention, or rectal incontinence.[67] Urinary retention precedes urinary incontinence because of initial weakening of the detrusor muscle.[68]

Surgical Options

Although little debate exists on whether to perform surgery, there is no consensus on which procedure to perform. Traditionally, a wide decompression with unilateral or bilateral laminectomy has been recommended and reported in the literature.[69,70] One recent study shows complete laminectomy is not required to adequately decompress the cauda equina.[71]

Timing of Surgery

The study by Kotsuik and colleagues[69] in 1986 is often quoted for the timing of surgical intervention. This retrospective review found that patients did not need surgical intervention within 6 hours of presentation. Although this is ideal, the ability to operate within 6 hours is difficult, if not impossible. The investigators did recommend operating within 48 hours but noted that the severity of symptoms were more important to long-term outcome than timing of surgery. Shapiro's original study[70] demonstrated that patients who had surgery within 48 hours had better outcomes than those who had surgery after 48 hours. The investigators did not recommend waiting the full 48 hours if it was possible to operate earlier. A later study by the same primary author showed that 24 hours was an "achievable and desirable goal."[68] A meta-analysis in 2000 showed statistical significance in patients treated within 48 hours versus those treated after 48 hours.[72]

Outcomes

Several major studies have reviewed outcomes in cauda equina. Shapiro's study looked at several outcomes, some of which significantly improved with surgery occurring within 48 hours. Nine of 13 patients recovered urologic function within 1 year, including all 7 who underwent surgery within 48 hours. Of the 7 who were sexually active and had sexual dysfunction, 5 recovered sexual function, including all 3 who underwent surgery within 48 hours. Chronic back pain was equal between both groups. One of 7 in the early operative group and 2 of 7 in the late operative group had chronic sciatica.[70]

Buchner and Schiltenwolf[73] also evaluated functional outcomes but did not relate them to timing of surgery. Seventeen of 22 regained complete urologic function, and 13 of 17 recovered motor function. Meanwhile, 21 patients had decreased sensation and 14 recovered the sensation; 87% of patients regained sensation in the perianal region.

In the meta-analysis by Ahn, and colleagues,[72] the investigators found similar results: 84% of patients had pain relief, and 75% regained motor function; sexual function returned in 67%, and 73% had urinary continence after losing it before surgery; only 56% regained sensory function, whereas 64% no longer had rectal incontinence.

SUMMARY

More than 75 years have passed since Mixter and Barr described surgical intervention for lumbar disk herniation. Although many questions have been answered regarding the surgical management of lumbar disk herniation, great debate still exists on which treatment provides the best outcomes. Surgical intervention seems to provide better outcomes when compared with nonsurgical management in patients with correlating radiologic and clinical findings who have failed an appropriate 4- to 6-week conservative management plan. No consensus exists as to which surgical approach provides the best results, but some evidence suggests that microsurgical and endoscopic techniques may cause less morbidity when compared with more traditional open techniques. Leg pain is more reliably relieved when compared with back pain, but prospective studies show some improvement in back pain in addition to leg pain. Surgery is fairly safe and has few major complications.

Cauda equina syndrome is a surgical urgency with decompression required as soon as possible. Patients have improved outcomes when decompression is performed within 48 hours and when their symptoms are less severe on presentation. More often than not, symptoms resolve, but sensory function less reliably resolves with pain typically improving.

REFERENCES

1. Mixter WJ, Barr JS. Rupture of the intervertebral disc with involvement of the spinal canal. N Engl J Med 1934;211:210–4.
2. Love JG. Removal of protruded intervertebral disc without laminectomy. Proc Staff Meet Mayo Clin 1939;14:32.
3. Semmes RE. Diagnosis of ruptured intervertebral disc without contrast myelography and comment upon recent experience with modified hemilaminectomy for their removal. Yale J Biol Med 1939;11(5):433.
4. Smith L. Enzyme dissolution of the nucleus pulposus in humans. J Am Med Assoc 1964;187(2):137.
5. Caspar W. A new surgical procedure for lumbar disc herniation causing less tissue damage through a microsurgical approach. Adv Neurosurg 1977; 4(74–9):152.
6. Yasargil MG. Microsurgical operation of herniated lumbar disc. Adv Neurosurg 1977;4:81.
7. Williams W. Microlumbar discectomy: a conservative surgical approach to the virgin herniated lumbar disc. Spine 1978;3(2):175.
8. Forst R, Hausmann B. Nucleoscopy: —a new examination technique. Arch Orthop Trauma Surg 1983;101(3):219–21.
9. Foley KT, Smith MM, Rampersaud YR. Microendoscopic discectomy. Tech Neurosurg 1997;3(4):301–7.
10. Bell GR, Rothman RH. The conservative treatment of sciatica. Spine 1984;9(1):54.
11. Hirsch C, Jonsson B, Lewin T. Low-back symptoms in a Swedish female population. Clin Orthop Relat Res 1969;63:171.
12. Dagenais S, Caro J, Haldeman S. A systematic review of low back pain cost of illness studies in the United States and internationally. Spine J 2008;8:8–20.
13. Weber H. Lumbar disc herniation: a controlled, prospective study with 10 years of observation. Spine 1983;8(2):131–40.
14. Atlas SJ, Deyo RA, Keller RB, et al. The Maine Lumbar Spine Study, Part II: 1-year outcomes of surgical and nonsurgical management of sciatica. Spine 1996; 21(15):1777.
15. Atlas SJ, Keller RB, Chang YC, et al. Surgical and nonsurgical management of sciatica secondary to a lumbar disc herniation: five-year outcomes from the Maine Lumbar Spine Study. Spine 2001;26(10):1179.
16. Atlas SJ, Keller RB, Wu YA, et al. Long-term outcomes of surgical and nonsurgical management of sciatica secondary to a lumbar disc herniation: 10 year results from the Maine Lumbar Spine Study. Spine 2005;30(8):927.
17. Weinstein JN, Tosteson TD, Lurie JD, et al. Surgical vs nonoperative treatment for lumbar disk herniation: the Spine Patient Outcomes Research Trial (SPORT): a randomized trial. J Am Med Assoc 2006;296(20):2441.
18. Weinstein JN, Lurie JD, Tosteson TD, et al. Surgical versus non-operative treatment for lumbar disc herniation: four-year results for the Spine Patient Outcomes Research Trial (SPORT). Spine 2008;33(25):2789.
19. Rydevik B, Brown MD, Lundborg G. Pathoanatomy and pathophysiology of nerve root compression. Spine 1984;9(1):7.
20. Gelfan S, Tarlov IM. Physiology of spinal cord, nerve root and peripheral nerve compression. Am J Physiol 1956;185(1):217.

21. Sharpless SK. Susceptibility of spinal roots to compression block. The research status of spinal manipulative therapy: a workshop held at the National Institutes of Health. February 2–4, Bethesda (MD): US Department of Health, Education, and Welfare, Public Health Service, National Institutes of Health, National Institute of Neurological and Communicative Disorders and Stroke; 1975. p. 155.
22. Olmarker K, Rydevik B, Holm S. Edema formation in spinal nerve roots induced by experimental, graded compression: an experimental study on the pig cauda equina with special reference to differences in effects between rapid and slow onset of compression. Spine 1989;14(6):569.
23. Olmarker K, Rydevik B, Hansson T, et al. Compression-induced changes of the nutritional supply to the porcine cauda equina. J Spinal Disord Tech 1990;3(1):25.
24. Olmarker K, Holm S, Rydevik B. Importance of compression onset rate for the degree of impairment of impulse propagation in experimental compression injury of the porcine cauda equina. Spine 1990;15(5):416.
25. Kuslich SD, Ulstrom CL, Michael CJ. The tissue origin of low back pain and sciatica: a report of pain response to tissue stimulation during operations on the lumbar spine using local anesthesia. Orthop Clin North Am 1991;22(2):181–7.
26. Olmarker K, Rydevik B, Nordborg C. Autologous nucleus pulposus induces neurophysiologic and histologic changes in porcine cauda equina nerve roots. Spine 1993;18(11):1425.
27. Olmarker K, Nordborg C, Larsson K, et al. Ultrastructural changes in spinal nerve roots induced by autologous nucleus pulposus. Spine 1996;21(4):411.
28. Olmarker K, Blomquist J, Strömberg J, et al. Inflammatogenic properties of nucleus pulposus. Spine 1995;20(6):665.
29. Olmarker K, Larsson K. Tumor necrosis factor alpha and nucleus-pulposus-induced nerve root injury. Spine 1998;23(23):2538.
30. Olmarker K, Rydevik B. Selective inhibition of tumor necrosis factor-alpha prevents nucleus pulposus-induced thrombus formation, intraneural edema, and reduction of nerve conduction velocity: possible implications for future pharmacologic treatment strategies of sciatica. Spine 2001;26(8):863.
31. Korhonen T, Karppinen J, Paimela L, et al. The treatment of disc herniation-induced sciatica with infliximab: results of a randomized, controlled, 3-month follow-up study. Spine 2005;30(24):2724.
32. Genevay S, Stingelin S, Gabay C. Efficacy of etanercept in the treatment of acute, severe sciatica: a pilot study. Ann Rheum Dis 2004;63(9):1120.
33. Bozzao A, Gallucci M, Masciocchi C, et al. Lumbar disk herniation: MR imaging assessment of natural history in patients treated without surgery. Radiology 1992;185(1):135.
34. Saal JA, Saal JS. Nonoperative treatment of herniated lumbar intervertebral disc with radiculopathy: an outcome study. Spine 1989;14(4):431.
35. Abumi K, Panjabi MM, Kramer KM, et al. Biomechanical evaluation of lumbar spinal stability after graded facetectomies. Spine 1990;15(11):1142.
36. Pintar FA, Cusick JF, Yoganandan N, et al. The biomechanics of lumbar facetectomy under compression-flexion. Spine 1992;17(7):804.
37. Haher TR, O'Brien M, Dryer JW, et al. The role of the lumbar facet joints in spinal stability: identification of alternative paths of loading. Spine 1994;19(23):2667.
38. Wilson DH, Harbaugh R. Microsurgical and standard removal of the protruded lumbar disc: a comparative study. Neurosurgery 1981;8(4):422–7.
39. Maroon JC, Abla AA. Microlumbar discectomy. Clin Neurosurg 1986;33:407.
40. Goald HJ. Microlumbar discectomy: followup of 147 patients. Spine 1978;3(2):183.

41. Nakagawa H, Kamimura M, Uchiyama S, et al. Microendoscopic discectomy (MED) for lumbar disc prolapse. J Clin Neurosci 2003;10(2):231–5.
42. Brayda-Bruno M, Cinnella P, Center SS, et al. Posterior endoscopic discectomy (and other procedures). Eur Spine J 2000;9:24–9.
43. Muramatsu K, Hachiya Y, Morita C. Postoperative magnetic resonance imaging of lumbar disc herniation: comparison of microendoscopic discectomy and Love's method. Spine 2001;26(14):1599.
44. Righesso O, Falavigna A, Avanzi O. Comparison of open discectomy with micro-endoscopic discectomy in lumbar disc herniations: results of a randomized controlled trial. Neurosurgery 2007;61(3):545.
45. Brock M, Kunkel P, Papavero L. Lumbar microdiscectomy: subperiosteal versus transmuscular approach and influence on the early postoperative analgesic consumption. Eur Spine J 2008;17(4):518–22.
46. Arts MP, Brand R, van den Akker ME, et al. Tubular diskectomy vs conventional microdiskectomy for sciatica: a randomized controlled trial. J Am Med Assoc 2009;302(2):149.
47. Fisher CG, Vaccaro AR, Thomas KC, et al. Evidence-based recommendations for spine surgery. Spine 2010;35(15):E678.
48. Wiese M, Krämer J, Bernsmann K, et al. The related outcome and complication rate in primary lumbar microscopic disc surgery depending on the surgeon's experience: comparative studies* 1. Spine J 2004;4(5):550–6.
49. Swartz KR, Trost GR. Recurrent lumbar disc herniation. Neurosurg Focus 2003;15(3):1–4.
50. Carragee EJ, Han MY, Suen PW, et al. Clinical outcomes after lumbar discectomy for sciatica: the effects of fragment type and anular competence. J Bone Joint Surg Am 2003;85(1):102.
51. Suk KS, Lee HM, Moon SH, et al. Recurrent lumbar disc herniation: results of operative management. Spine 2001;26(6):672.
52. Carragee EJ, Spinnickie AO, Alamin TF, et al. A prospective controlled study of limited versus subtotal posterior discectomy: short-term outcomes in patients with herniated lumbar intervertebral discs and large posterior anular defect. Spine 2006;31(6):653.
53. Barth M, Diepers M, Weiss C, et al. Two-year outcome after lumbar microdiscectomy versus microscopic sequestrectomy: part 2: radiographic evaluation and correlation with clinical outcome. Spine 2008;33(3):273.
54. Ammerman JM, Ammerman MD, Dambrosia J, et al. A prospective evaluation of the role for intraoperative x-ray in lumbar discectomy. Predictors of incorrect level exposure. Surg Neurol 2006;66(5):470–3.
55. Davis RA. A long-term outcome analysis of 984 surgically treated herniated lumbar discs. J Neurosurg 1994;80(3):415–21.
56. Toyone T, Tanaka T, Kato D, et al. Low-back pain following surgery for lumbar disc herniation. A prospective study. J Bone Joint Surg Am 2004;86(5):893.
57. Asch HL, Lewis PJ, Moreland DB, et al. Prospective multiple outcomes study of outpatient lumbar microdiscectomy: should 75 to 80% success rates be the norm? J Neurosurg 2002;96(1):34–44.
58. Hanley EN, Shapiro DE. The development of low-back pain after excision of a lumbar disc. J Bone Joint Surg Am 1989;71(5):719.
59. Haddad GH. Analysis of 2932 workers' compensation back injury cases: the impact on the cost to the system. Spine 1987;12(8):765.
60. Greenough CG, Fraser RD. The effects of compensation on recovery from low-back injury. Spine 1989;14(9):947.

61. Sander RA, Meyers JE. The relationship of disability to compensation status in railroad workers. Spine 1986;11(2):141.
62. Lurie JD, Faucett SC, Hanscom B, et al. Lumbar discectomy outcomes vary by herniation level in the spine patient outcomes research trial. J Bone Joint Surg Am 2008;90(9):1811.
63. Österman H, Seitsalo S, Karppinen J, et al. Effectiveness of microdiscectomy for lumbar disc herniation: a randomized controlled trial with 2 years of follow-up. Spine 2006;31(21):2409.
64. Spangfort EV. The lumbar disc herniation. A computer-aided analysis of 2,504 operations. Acta Orthop Scand Suppl 1972;142:1.
65. Loupasis GA, Stamos K, Katonis PG, et al. Seven-to 20-year outcome of lumbar discectomy. Spine 1999;24(22):2313.
66. Spector LR, Madigan L, Rhyne A, et al. Cauda equina syndrome. J Am Acad Orthop Surg 2008;16(8):471.
67. Domen PM, Hofman PA, van Santbrink H, et al. Predictive value of clinical characteristics in patients with suspected cauda equina syndrome. Eur J Neurol 2009;16(3):416–9.
68. Shapiro S. Medical realities of cauda equina syndrome secondary to lumbar disc herniation. Spine 2000;25(3):348–51 [discussion: 352].
69. Kostuik JP, Harrington I, Alexander D, et al. Cauda equina syndrome and lumbar disc herniation. J Bone Joint Surg Am 1986;68(3):386.
70. Shapiro S. Cauda equina syndrome secondary to lumbar disc herniation. Neurosurgery 1993;32(5):743.
71. Olivero WC, Wang H, Hanigan WC, et al. Cauda equina syndrome (CES) from lumbar disc herniations. J Spinal Disord Tech 2009;22(3):202–6.
72. Ahn UM, Ahn NU, Buchowski JM, et al. Cauda equina syndrome secondary to lumbar disc herniation: a meta-analysis of surgical outcomes. Spine 2000; 25(12):1515.
73. Buchner M, Schiltenwolf M. Cauda equina syndrome caused by intervertebral lumbar disk prolapse: mid-term results of 22 patients and literature review. Orthopedics 2002;25(7):727–31.

Surgical Treatment and Outcomes of Cervical Radiculopathy

Robert C. Decker, MD

KEYWORDS

- Cervical radiculopathy • Arm pain
- Anterior cervical diskectomy (ACDF)
- Anterior cervical foraminotomy (ACF)
- Cervical disk replacement • Cervical disk arthroplasty (CDA)
- Posterior cervical foraminotomy (PCF)

Generally, neck pain and cervical radiculopathy is self-limiting, so ample time should be afforded to nonsurgical treatments. Lees and Turner[1] demonstrated a generally favorable course for cervical radiculopathy and found that 45% of patients had only a single episode of pain without recurrence and 30% had only mild symptoms. However, although most patients improved, the investigators found that 25% of patients had persistent or worsening symptoms. When nonoperative techniques, such as time, physical therapy, traction, and injections, fail to provide acceptable relief from symptoms, surgery may be required to address the pathologic condition causing pain.

The trajectory of cervical nerve roots from the spinal cord to the neuroforamen causes the root to be vulnerable to ventral pathologic conditions. Generally, pathologic conditions can be caused by a soft or hard disk. A soft disk occurs when a fragment of the nucleus pulposis herniates through the annulus, whereas a hard disk develops with time as osteophytes form in response to altered mechanics secondary to motion segment degeneration.[2]

SURGICAL INDICATIONS

Accepted surgical indications for cervical radiculopathy include severe or progressive neurologic deficit or significant pain that does not respond to appropriate

Disclosures: none.
Department of Orthopaedics and Rehabilitation, Orthopaedics & Sports Medicine Institute, University of Florida, 3450 Hull Road, Room 3341, Gainesville, FL 32607, USA
E-mail address: deckerc@ortho.ufl.edu

Phys Med Rehabil Clin N Am 22 (2011) 179–191
doi:10.1016/j.pmr.2010.12.001
1047-9651/11/$ – see front matter © 2011 Elsevier Inc. All rights reserved.

nonoperative treatments. Before surgical intervention, it is vital to correlate the anatomic distribution of signs and symptoms to radiographic images.

Mummaneni and colleagues[3] found that surgery had the greatest success when compression found on magnetic resonance imaging (MRI) correlated with the patient's signs and symptoms. Electromyography (EMG) demonstrated poor sensitivity in detecting cervical radiculopathy, so utility was mixed in predicting surgical outcomes. The investigators recommended EMG in patients with unusual or atypical symptoms or in those with multifocal causes.

Sasso and colleagues[4] evaluated selective nerve root injections (SNRIs) both in the cervical and lumbar spine to determine if they could predict surgical outcomes for radiculopathy. The investigators retrospectively reviewed 101 patients who had undergone SNRI and surgical decompression and found that 91% of patients with a good response to SNRI (good outcome occurred if there was greater than 95% pain relief) had good surgical outcomes (good surgical outcome was defined as a postoperative visual analog scale [VAS] ≤ 2 and a satisfied patient). Only 60% of the patients had a good surgical outcome when SNRI did not provide temporary symptomatic relief. The investigators also found that patients with a positive MRI finding had an 87% good surgical outcome, whereas patients with a negative MRI finding had a surgical success of 85%. When MRI and SNRI results conflicted, the SNRI results were more consistent with the surgical outcome. Lumbar and cervical cases were not individually reviewed, and with the associated risks of paralysis and stroke with cervical SNRI, injections in the cervical spine may be best suited for equivocal cases as long as the patient understands the risks. Overall, to provide the best possible outcome, the imaging interventions and the patient's signs and symptoms must correlate.

Many surgical options exist to address cervical radiculopathy. The offending pathologic condition can be addressed through an anterior or posterior approach. In addition, surgery can consist of simple decompression or decompression with a fusion or motion sparing device. This article describes numerous surgical techniques that are offered at present, reviews their respective indications, and examines their outcomes.

SURGICAL OPTIONS
Posterior Cervical Foraminotomy

Spurling and Scoville[5] initially described posterior decompression for cervical radicular pain in the 1940s, before the introduction of anterior decompression. The technique consisted of a cervical laminectomy followed by removal of the disk. This approach evolved into the posterior cervical foraminotomy (PCF) described by Frykholm[6] in the early 1950s, in which minimal bone is removed from the lamina and facet joint to decompress the exiting nerve root. The benefits of posterior decompression include direct visualization of the exiting nerve root and decompression without need for fusion and the resulting alteration of spinal kinematics. PCF is effective for posterolateral soft disk herniations as well as indirect decompression of neuroforaminal stenosis.

The patient's head is stabilized in the prone position, and the level of decompression is determined by fluoroscopy. Subperiosteal dissection is performed down to the lamina, with the muscular attachments cephalad and caudad to the targeted level, and the interspinous ligament is left intact. A hemilaminotomy is performed, with the lateral portions of the lamina and medial aspect of the facet joint burred down with a high-speed burr under microscopic or loupe visualization. The cervical facet joint must be partially removed to expose and decompress the nerve root. Once the nerve root is identified, any remaining compressive bony or ligamentous lesion is carefully removed. If additional room is required to remove a soft disk herniation, a portion of the pedicle can be resected.[7–10] The surgeon must be careful with the amount of facet joint removed, because removal of more than 50% of the facet results in significantly increased posterior strain and spinal instability and, therefore, should be avoided.[11]

Anterior Cervical Diskectomy and Fusion

Smith and Robinson[12] as well as Cloward[13] described the anterior cervical diskectomy and fusion (ACDF) in 1958, and at present, it is the most widely used surgical procedure for cervical radiculopathy. The benefit of the anterior approach is the removal of ventral compressive lesions without the need for retraction of the spinal cord. Smith and Robinson[12] advocated the removal of the disk and placement of an iliac crest bone autograft to encourage fusion. Osteophytes were not removed, because they were thought to resorb once a fusion was obtained and motion ceased. Cloward[13] described the procedure with the use of cylindrical bone dowels filled with morselized autograft.

ACDF is performed supine with a bump between the shoulder blades to place the neck in gentle extension. The incision is marked with fluoroscopy and landmarks. Dissection is carried down through the skin and subcutaneous tissue to the platysma fascia. The fascia is split longitudinally to expose the medial border of the sternocleidomastoid muscle. The carotid sheath is palpated laterally, and the anterior cervical spine is approached using blunt dissection through fascial planes. The precervical spinal fascia is divided, and the longus colli muscle is mobilized laterally after a lateral radiographic image verifies the correct level. The disk is first removed to decompress the spinal canal followed by any osteophytes. The neuroforamin and exiting nerve roots are probed with a micronerve hook to ensure adequate decompression.

After the neural elements are decompressed, attention is turned to preparing the spine for fusion and placing the interbody graft. Although fusion without an interbody is described in the literature, there has been a decrease in the amount of anterior diskectomies done without fusion, secondary to an increased incidence of neck pain and postoperative kyphosis.[14] An interbody graft assists with the expansion of the neuroforaminal space and it therefore provides indirect decompression of the nerve roots. There are multiple choices of interbody grafts, including autograft, allograft, and polyether ether ketone, that can be used. As the allograft has become more available, it has reduced the use of autograft bone because it does not have associated donor-site morbidity.[15,16]

In the 1990s, cervical plates were introduced to augment stability. The addition of a cervical plate may help decrease the risk of pseudoarthrosis, maintain lordosis, and decrease the need for postoperative bracing because of the greater stability offered. However, the plates have been associated with an increased risk of dysphagia and implant failure due to screw loosening and backing out.[15,17,18] Current plates are engineered to prevent screw back out, and thus this complication has been reduced.[19] When using autograft, plating does not change the fusion rate when a 1 level fusion is performed, although the plate may prevent segmental kyphosis and graft subsidence.[20] Plating does help increase the fusion rate when multiple levels are addressed, regardless of graft choice.[21–23]

Cervical Disk Arthroplasty

The risk of adjacent segment degeneration both above and below a fusion led to the development of technologies to preserve cervical motion. The theoretical benefit of cervical disk arthroplasty (CDA) is the maintenance of motion at the diseased level. Motion within normal physiologic ranges theoretically helps to decrease stress at adjacent segments as compared with fusion, which has been shown to increase adjacent disk stress.[24–28]

Numerous manufacturers have produced or are in the process of producing CDA devices. The Bryan cervical disc (Medtronic Sofamor Danek, Memphis, TN, USA) and the ProDisc-C (Synthes Spine Company, LP, West Chester, PA, USA) are 2 devices that have been through investigational device exemption (IDE) trials by the US Food and Drug Administration agency (FDA) to determine if equivalent performance exists with CDA compared with the ACDF, the current standard of care.

The surgical approach to the anterior cervical spine is the same as that for ACDF. Once the disk is removed and the neurologic structures are decompressed, the cartilaginous end plates are removed, leaving the bony end plates of the vertebral bodies to provide a firm foundation for the implant. A wider decompression is necessary because motion is preserved so that osteophytes may reform. A distracter is used to recreate the normal disk height, and trial devices are inserted to properly size the implant. The vertebral bodies are prepared as directed by the individual characteristics of the implant and then the implant is inserted and final implant positioning is confirmed with imaging. Patients undergoing CDA may receive antiinflammatory medication to decrease postoperative pain as well as potentially decrease the risk of heterotypic bone ossification. Because CDA hopes to maintain motion at the segment, the risk of pseudoarthrosis is eliminated, and this technique may help to decrease the risk of adjacent segment degeneration.

Anterior Cervical Foraminotomy

More recently, an anterior cervical foraminotomy (ACF) has been described to directly decompress the nerve root without fusion. Through this approach, a posterolateral disk herniation or foraminal stenosis can be addressed. Patient history, examination, and advanced imaging should all point to a well-defined anatomic site of unilateral nerve impingement. Patients should have predominant arm pain, because neck pain is a poor surgical indication.[29–31] The approach is similar to that described for an ACDF, except the longus colli muscle is incised and kept lateral to expose the lateral disk and uncovertebral joint. Synder and Bernhardt[32] first described a limited anterior foraminotomy, in which the lateral third of the disk was removed and the uncovertebral joint resected to decompress the nerve root. To improve outcomes and maintain the disk's integrity, Jho[29] altered the technique to leave as much of the disk intact, while removing the entire uncovertebral joint to decompress the nerve root. In this technique, the vertebral artery was exposed, which carried a risk of iatrogenic injury. Saringer and colleagues[31] modified Jho's technique by leaving the lateral wall of the uncovertebral joint intact during burring to protect the vertebral artery. Through this approach, they were still able to decompress the nerve root from its origin at the spinal cord to the point where it passes posterior to the vertebral artery. More recently, Lee and colleagues[30] modified the technique by burring from the base of the uncinate process, leaving the intervertebral space intact. The uncinate process is not completely resected, and the investigators assert that the functional anatomy remains intact with no evidence of delayed instability in clinical follow-up.

OUTCOMES
PCF Outcomes

PCF has demonstrated excellent results when performed for the correct indications while maintaining motion at the diseased vertebral segment. In a retrospective study, Henderson and colleagues[33] reported good to excellent results in 91.5% of 846 patients, with resolution of radicular symptoms and motor deficits in 96% and 98%, respectively. Complications such as wound infection and dehiscence were observed in 1.5%, while a radiculopathy recurrence rate of 3.5% was demonstrated. They recommended PCF for simple cervical radicular problems. Tomaras and colleagues[34] observed similar results in a review of 182 patients who underwent PCF and found that 93% of patients had a good to excellent result after a mean of 19 months.

Jagannathan and colleagues,[8] in a recent retrospective review of 162 single-level PCFs performed for unilateral radiculopathy, concluded that the procedure was highly successful. About 93% of patients had an improvement in their neck disability index (NDI), and 95% had resolution of radicular symptoms. These outcomes were maintained at a mean follow-up of 77 months.

Tumialan and colleagues,[35] in a retrospective review of military personnel with unilateral cervical radiculopathy, found that posterior foraminotomy offered a significant cost benefit compared with ACDF in both the short- and long-term. This advantage was secondary to patients not requiring instrumentation and interbody grafts. No significant difference was observed in the success of the procedures, defined as a return to active duty, but the patients who underwent PCF were able to return to active duty faster and at a lower cost.

Although PCF provides excellent results in the proper patient, risks exist. A radiographic review at a mean of 77 months by Jagannathan and colleagues[8] demonstrated no significant changes in either focal or segmental kyphosis and no changes in disk space height. However, loss of lordosis (defined by Cobb angle <10°) was observed in 20% of patients and represented the most common complication in Jagannathan's series. Although there was no significant risk for worsening of kyphosis in the general population, some patient subsets demonstrated loss of lordosis. Risk factors for worsening of sagittal alignment were age greater than 60 years at the time of the initial surgery, preoperative loss of lordosis, and need for further posterior surgery after the initial foraminotomy.[8] The extent of decompression, violation of the posterior muscular and ligamentous tension band, and resection of the facet joints all play a role in the loss of cervical alignment.

Although ACDF is associated with adjacent segment degeneration, it also occurs with PCF. Clarke and colleagues[36] reviewed 303 patients who underwent single-level PCF and found that the 10-year risk of adjacent segment degeneration was 6.7%. Jagannathan and colleagues,[8] at 8-year follow-up, found adjacent segment degeneration in 4.9% of patients, with a risk of developing it being 1.2% per year. These rates are less than those found in ACDF, as observed in the study by Hilibrand and colleagues[37] on adjacent segment degeneration after ACDF.

In addition to kyphosis and adjacent segment degeneration, postoperative instability was found in 4.9% of patients in the series by Jagannathan and colleagues,[8] but only 1 of 8 patients was symptomatic requiring fusion. Other complications included cerebrospinal fluid leak in 2.5% and C5 nerve root injury in 1.2% of the patients. In other series, nerve root injuries have been described in as many as 10% of the patients.[10]

Woertgen and colleagues,[38] in a prospective consecutive study of 54 patients who underwent PCF, found that a long duration of symptoms and neurologic deficits were important prognostic factors for a poor outcome. Also, patients with neck pain do not respond as well to PCF.[8] Overall, PCF is good procedure with excellent results when performed in the patient with the proper indications.

ACF Outcomes

Outcome data for ACF are limited to a small number of short-term follow-up studies reviewing multiple technique variations. Snyder and Bernhardt[32] reviewed 63 patients at a mean follow-up of 23 months and found that 64% of the patients had a good to excellent outcome, whereas more than one-third of the patients had either a fair or poor outcome. The technique of Snyder and Bernhardt[32] involved removing some of the disk and retaining some of the uncovertebral joint, which may have left residual compression and destabilized the joint. On an average, patients lost 1 mm of disk height, and 4% went on to experience spontaneous fusion. Despite this consequence, 85% of the patients were satisfied by their results. Hacker and Miller,[39] in a retrospective review of 23 patients who underwent ACF, found that 52% had a good to excellent outcome, whereas 30% required an additional procedure. The investigators raised issue over the number of poor results and the increased reoperation rate compared with other cervical radiculopathy treatments. These rates may be due to the development of postoperative spinal instability at the operated level.

Although the 2 previous studies demonstrated negative results, several studies have demonstrated positive findings. Johnson and colleagues,[40] using Jho's technique of not violating the disk, retrospectively reviewed 21 patients treated with ACF. They found that 91% of the patients either had improved or resolved radicular symptoms. No evidence of spinal instability in flexion or extension was observed at the short-term follow-up of 3 months of the studies. Saringer and colleagues[31] reviewed 34 patients with 2 to 17 months of follow-up and determined that 97% of patients had improvement in both neck pain and radicular symptoms. Paresis and numbness improved in most patients but took longer. Equal success was observed in both 1 and 2 level decompressions. Lee and colleagues[30] reviewed 13 patients followed up for a mean of 19 months, with all patients getting 100% relief from radicular symptoms without evidence of instability. VAS score improved from 9.6 preoperatively to 2 postoperatively, with NDI score improvement from 41 to 16.

Similar to PCF's problem with excessive facet joint resection, unilateral uncovertebral joint resection can affect the stability of the spinal motion segment.[41–43] Chen and colleagues[42] demonstrated that resection of the unilateral uncovertebral joint alters normal spinal motion. Kotani and colleagues[43] sequentially resected different portions of the uncovertebral joint and found that the foraminal segment, resected with ACF, contributed the most to spinal segment stability. In addition, they demonstrated that uncovertebral joint resection resulted in a decreased overall stability of the spinal segment. No long-term studies exist as they do for ACDF evaluating the effect of ACF on the motion segment, disk degeneration, and adjacent segment degeneration.

Although the studies reviewing ACF have demonstrated mostly positive results, several questions exist. Hacker and Miller[39] specifically raised issue with the results of ACF and did not recommend the procedure as a stand-alone treatment for cervical radiculopathy. Overall, the studies do not present long-term results and represent several different technique variations. Further long-term data are needed to shed light on the viability of ACF.

ACDF Outcomes

ACDF has been used for many decades with good results in treating cervical radiculopathy. White and colleagues[44] demonstrated good to excellent results in 76% of patients who underwent ACDF for radicular symptoms. They found that a successful fusion led to better results. Bohlman and colleagues[45] reviewed the outcomes of 122 patients who underwent 1 to 4 level ACDF with autogenous iliac crest bone graft, with an average follow-up of 6 years. They demonstrated that 93% of patients had no pain or only mild pain and were considered good to excellent outcomes. Of the 122 patients, 55 had neurologic deficits preoperatively and all but 2 had complete resolution of their symptoms. They determined that overall, ACDF was a safe procedure that can relieve pain and lead to a resolution of neurologic symptoms in a large percentage of patients.

Recently, good outcome data regarding ACDF have been published from the randomized controlled multicenter clinical trials evaluating CDA, in which ACDF was used as the control. Heller and colleagues[25] demonstrated that ACDF caused a significant reduction in arm and neck pain from preoperative values. A 15-point reduction in the NDI was demonstrated with a 1 level ACDF, with maintenance or improvement of neurologic status in 90.2% of patients. In addition, significant improvement was observed in the 36-Item Short Form Health Survey (SF-36) scores, mental health scores, as well as in NDI scores. Improvements in SF-36 scores after ACDF were found to be greater than or equal to the improvement observed after total knee and hip arthroplasty. Radiographic evaluation identified a nonunion rate of roughly 6% in the 1 level ACDF with an allograft spacer and plate at 24 months. Results were maintained at 2-year follow-up. Overall, when looking at multiple variables with a 1 level ACDF, success was observed in 72.7% of patients.

The study by Murrey and colleagues[16] on CDA also demonstrated good results after ACDF. About 78% of patients who underwent 1 level ACDF had a successful reduction of their neck disability (success was characterized by the FDA as a 15-point improvement in NDI) and improvement in SF-36 scores. Neurologic success rate, defined as maintenance or improvement of neurologic function, was observed at 2-year follow-up in 88% of patients who underwent ACDF. About 83% of patients who underwent ACDF were completely satisfied, with 80.9% stating that they would undergo the procedure again. Fusion rate was determined to be 90.2% at 24 months, and 8.5% of patients who underwent ACDF required a secondary surgical procedure within the follow-up period. There was a significant improvement at all time points for the ACDF population in SF-36 score improvement from baseline. Overall, success was observed in 68.3% of patients who underwent fusion, when all the FDA-defined criteria were composited.[16]

Although ACDF has been performed for many years and has demonstrated good overall outcomes and low morbidity, risks exist. They include dysphagia (up to 60%),[46] dysphonia (up to 51%),[46] injury to the esophagus, pseudoarthrosis, and hardware failure.[21,45,47,48] Morbidity can be affected by several different variables, such as smoking history, number of levels fused, plating, and type of graft used.[45,47] There is an increased risk of dysphagia and dysphonia in patients who have preoperative complaints of these conditions before surgery. In addition, patients with gastroesophageal reflux disease also have an increased risk of postoperative complaints with breathing, voice, and swallowing and they should be counseled appropriately.[46]

Bohlman and colleagues[45] found that pseudoarthrosis risk increased with the number of levels treated and that there was a significant association between postoperative pain and pseudoarthrosis. Zdeblick and colleagues[49] demonstrated that reoperation for symptomatic pseudoarthrosis or persistent symptoms after ACDF can lead to excellent outcomes, as shown by 83% of patients after revision.

An additional risk associated with ACDF is adjacent segment degeneration leading to a return or development of new symptoms.[50] Adjacent segment degeneration has been reported to occur in 3% to 8% of patients per year as a consequence of ACDF.[16,37,51–54] Hilibrand and colleagues[37] determined that adjacent segment degeneration occurred at a relatively constant incidence of 2.9% per year for the first 10 years after cervical arthrodesis. In addition, survivorship analysis predicted that 25.6% of patients would have new degeneration within 10 years. This degeneration is believed to be secondary to genetics, the natural progression of cervical disease, and increased stress at adjacent levels after fusion due to altered spinal kinematics.[28,55,56] Hilibrand and colleagues[37] found that adjacent degeneration was less likely after a multilevel fusion when compared with a single-level fusion.

CDA Outcomes

Although the studies on CDA provide a good indication of ACDF success rate, they primarily provide information on the CDA and its comparison to ACDF. Heller and colleagues,[25] in a prospective randomized clinical IDE trial, examined the results of the Bryan cervical disc and ACDF (control) at 2-year follow-up. The indication for surgery was radiculopathy or myelopathy in patients with single-level cervical pathologic condition. At 2-year follow-up, the radiographic range of motion was $8.1° \pm 4.8°$ in the investigational group, demonstrating continued segment motion. The artificial disk group had a statistically superior improvement in NDI compared with ACDF group and an overall higher rate of overall success at 2 years. Overall success was measured with a composite score comprised of clinical and safety outcomes. Although arm pain reduction and SF-36 scores were similar in both groups, the arthroplasty group demonstrated a significantly greater improvement in neck pain at all time points. Patients who underwent arthroplasty returned to work 13 days earlier than those who underwent fusion, which was statistically significant. No difference was observed in adverse events between ACDF and CDA. Overall, cervical disk replacement was recommended as a viable alternative to ACDF.[25]

Murrey and colleagues[16] reported on the 2-year data from 209 patients in the FDA IDE study of the ProDisc-C. There were no differences observed between CDA and ACDF regarding neck and arm VAS scores, NDI, SF-36, or neurologic status at 24 months. Although there was a significantly increased operative time (8.5 minutes) and blood loss (20 mL) with arthroplasty, the arthroplasty group demonstrated a decreased reoperation rate (1.8% vs 8.5%) as compared with ACDF. The IDE study by Murrey and colleagues[16] demonstrated that the CDA was safe and effective at 24 months compared with ACDF.

To date, the US multicenter CDA IDE studies have only released their 2-year cumulative results, with longer follow-up expected. However, Garrido and colleagues[57] reviewed the 48-month data from a single institution involved in the prospective Bryan IDE trial and demonstrated no decrease in the outcomes for arm or neck VAS, NDI, or SF-36 compared with ACDF at 4 years. In addition, patients who underwent CDA continued to require less number of secondary surgeries.

Goffin and colleagues[58] published longer-term observational results of CDA from a multicenter European study evaluating arthroplasty using Bryan cervical disc in 98 patients (89 [1 level] and 9 [2 level]) without a control group. CDA was performed for radiculopathy or myelopathy associated with spondylosis and/or disk herniations unresponsive to conservative treatment. The investigators found the favorable clinical outcomes noted at 2 years were maintained at the intermediate time points of 4 to 6 years. SF-36, NDI, and neck and arm pain results were all improved compared with preoperative values and maintained over the course of the study. Motion was maintained within 2° of the preoperative value in more than 83% of patients who underwent 1 level arthroplasty demonstrating motion greater than 2° (2° was the cut-off point for showing motion existed). Although motion existed, it was decreased at the 4- and 6-year follow-up as compared with the 1- and 2-year time points. Only 5.8% of patients experienced adverse events secondary to the arthroplasty device. Overall, the favorable clinical and angular motion outcomes that were noted at 1- and 2-year follow-up persist at 4- and 6-year follow-up.[58] Time will determine if this finding holds true for the more rigorous US FDA studies.

CDA shares the same surgical approach with ACDF, and many of the surgical risks are similar. Anderson and colleagues[59] reviewed the adverse events that occurred during the Bryan IDE study at 24 months. There were no significant differences in the overall medical events between CDA and ACDF. Although the CDA group had more surgically related adverse events than the ACDF group, they tended to be less severe, such as dysphagia or late medical events. Overall, although the ACDF group had fewer events, the events were more severe because of the treatment of pseudoarthrosis and persistent symptoms requiring a higher rate of reoperation. Both procedures were demonstrated to be safe, with overall low incidences of adverse events.

Walraevens and colleagues,[60] in a prospective longitudinal study, found that mobility at the CDA-treated level was preserved in 85% or more of the 84 patients studied at 8-year follow-up. Although increased segmental motion was not observed at adjacent levels, disk degeneration increased at adjacent levels, a condition CDA attempts to mitigate. The increase in degeneration at adjacent levels was commensurate to disk degeneration observed in natural age-related studies and less than that found in ACDF studies. Radiographic evidence of heterotopic ossification was found in up to 39% of patients at the treated level within the first 4 years and remained stable beyond that. No patient exhibited anteroposterior device migration or subsidence. CDA maintains preoperative motion at the index and adjacent levels and seems to protect against acceleration of adjacent-level degeneration as is often observed later.

Recently, CDA is being used by combining it with fusion or above or below a previous fusion. Barbagallo and colleagues[61] reported on using a hybrid of CDA and fusion for patients with multilevel disease in 2 level, 3 level, and 4 level surgeries. They found it to be safe and reliable, with good maintenance of results with follow-up of 12 to 40 months. In addition, Phillips and colleagues[18] observed single-level CDA adjacent to prior ACDF compared with CDA in patients without previous fusion. They found that both groups demonstrated significant improvement in NDI and VAS after surgery, without significant difference between the 2 groups. Despite increased biomechanical forces at the level adjacent due to fusion, CDA did well in the short-term, although longer-term follow-up is required.

Comparison of Anterior and Posterior Procedures

The literature contains few studies that review both anterior decompression with ACDF and posterior decompression with PCF. Herkowitz and colleagues[62] prospectively reviewed 33 patients who underwent treatment of posterolateral cervical soft disk herniations with either an anterior (ACDF) or posterior (PCF) approach. About 94% of patients who underwent ACDF had a good to excellent result, whereas 75% who underwent PCF had similar results. Onimus and colleagues[63] reviewed anterior and posterior decompression for soft posterolateral cervical disk herniations, with similar results between the 2 groups.

In well-selected patients with unilateral radiculopathy, decompression of the lateral recess and neuroforamin by either ACDF or posterior foraminotomy has been found to be efficacious. Additional studies using current treatment options, including CDA and minimally invasive PCF, would be beneficial in determining the ideal approach. Trends in the United States over the past few decades have shifted in favor of an anterior approach.[64,65] However, it has been recently suggested that PCF may play a larger role in the future with the introduction of newer minimally invasive techniques and the decreased cost and risks due to not needing instrumentation and fusion.[35,66]

SUMMARY

Cervical radiculopathy, although generally self-limiting, can be resistant to conservative treatment requiring surgical treatment. Care must be taken to determine the source and level of the source of the pathologic condition to maximize postoperative results. At present, both ACDF and PCF are good treatment options in the suitable patient. ACF has not shown the same success, and long-term studies of a large group of patients are lacking at present. In general, the potential morbidity of the procedures should be matched to the patient's symptoms to best choose the surgical approach and plan that offers the greatest chance of long-term relief. CDA may show benefit to ACDF in the future, but long-term outcomes from the US FDA studies are still pending and will prove interesting to review.

REFERENCES

1. Lees F, Turner JW. Natural history and prognosis of cervical spondylosis. Br Med J 1963;2:1607–10.
2. Emery SE, Bohlman HH. Osteoarthritis of the C-spine. Chapter 30. In: Moskowitz RW, Howell DS, Goldberg VM, et al, editors. Osteoarthritis, diagnosis and management. 2nd edition. Philadelphia: WB Saunders Co; 1992. p. 651–68.
3. Mummaneni PV, Kaiser MG, Matz PG, et al. Preoperative patient selection with magnetic resonance imaging, computer tomography and electroencephalography: does the test predict outcome after cervical surgery? J Neurosurg Spine 2009;11:119–29.
4. Sasso RC, Macadaeg K, Nordmann D, et al. Selective nerve root injections can predict surgical outcome for lumbar and cervical radiculopathy; comparison to magnetic resonance imaging. J Spinal Disord Tech 2005;18:471–8.
5. Spurling RG, Scoville WB. Lateral rupture of the cervical intervertebral disks: a common cause of shoulder and arm pain. Surg Gynecol Obstet 1944;78: 350–8.
6. Frykholm R. Cervical root compression resulting from disc degeneration and root sleeve fibrosis. Acta Chir Scand 1951;160:1–149.
7. Fessler RG, Khoo LT. Minimally invasive cervical microendoscopic foraminotomy, an initial clinical experience. Neurosurgery 2002;51:S37–45.
8. Jagannathan J, Sherman JH, Szabo T, et al. The posterior cervical foraminotomy in the treatment of cervical disc/osteophyte disease: a single-surgeon experience with a minimum of 5 years clinical and radiographic follow-up. J Neurosurg Spine 2009;10:347–56.
9. O'Toole JE, Sheikh H, Eichholz KM, et al. Endoscopic posterior cervical foraminotomy and discectomy. Neurosurg Clin N Am 2006;17:411–22.
10. Williams RW. Microsurgical foraminotomy. A surgical alternative for intractable radicular pain. Spine 1983;8:708–16.
11. Zdeblick TA, Zou D, Warden KE, et al. Cervical stability after foraminotomy. A biomechanical in vitro analysis. J Bone Joint Surg Am 1992;74:22–7.
12. Smith GW, Robinson RA. The treatment of certain cervical spine disorders by anterior removal of the intervertebral disc and interbody fusion. J Bone Joint Surg Am 1958;40:607–24.
13. Cloward RB. The anterior approach for removal of ruptured cervical discs. J Neurosurg 1958;15:602–17.
14. Watters WC III, Levinthal R. Anterior cervical discectomy with and without fusion: results, complications, and long-term follow-up. Spine 1994;19:2343–7.

15. Kaiser MG, Haid RW Jr, Subach BR, et al. Anterior cervical plating enhances arthrodesis after discectomy and fusion with cortical allograft. Neurosurgery 2002;50:229–36.
16. Murrey D, Janssen M, Delamarter R, et al. Results of the prospective, random-ized, controlled multicenter Food and Drug Administration Investigational Device Exemption study of the ProDisc-C total disc replacement versus anterior discec-tomy and fusion for the treatment of 1 level symptomatic cervical disc disease. Spine J 2009;9:275–86.
17. Fountas KN, Kapsalaki EZ, Nikolakakos LG, et al. Anterior cervical discectomy and fusion associated complications. Spine 2007;32:2310–7.
18. Phillips FM, Allen TR, Regan JJ, et al. Cervical disc replacement in patients with and without previous adjacent level fusion surgery: a prospective study. Spine 2009;34:556–65.
19. Geisler FH, Caspar W, Pitzen T, et al. Anterior cervical screw extrusion leading to acute upper airway obstruction: case report. Spine 2005;30:E683–6.
20. Wang JC, McDonough PW, Endow KK, et al. The effect of cervical plating on single-level anterior cervical discectomy and fusion. J Spinal Disord 1999;12: 467–71.
21. Samartzis D, Shen FH, Matthews DK, et al. Comparison of allograft to autograft in multilevel anterior cervical discectomy and fusion with rigid plate fixation. Spine J 2003;3:451–9.
22. Wang JC, McDonough PW, Endow KK, et al. Increased fusion rates with cervical plating for two-level anterior cervical discectomy and fusion. Spine 2000;25:41–5.
23. Wang JC, McDonough PW, Kamin LE, et al. Increased fusion rates with cervical plating for three-level anterior cervical discectomy and fusion. Spine 2001;26: 643–7.
24. DiAngelo DJ, Foley KT, Morrow BR, et al. In vitro biomechanics of cervical disc arthroplasty with the ProDisc-C total disc implant. Neurosurg Focus 2004;17:E4.
25. Heller JG, Sasso RC, Papadopoulos SM, et al. Comparison of Bryan cervical disc arthroplasty with anterior cervical decompression and fusion: clinical and radio-graphic results of a randomized, controlled, clinical trial. Spine 2009;34:101–7.
26. Mummaneni PV, Burkus JK, Haid RW, et al. Clinical and radiographic analysis of cervical disc arthroplasty compared with allograft fusion: a randomized controlled clinical trial. J Neurosurg Spine 2007;6:198–209.
27. Puttlitz CM, Rousseau MA, Xu Z, et al. Intervertebral disc replacement maintains cervical spine kinetics. Spine 2004;29:2809–14.
28. Reitman CA, Hipp JA, Nguyen L, et al. Changes in segmental intervertebral motion adjacent to cervical arthrodesis: a prospective study. Spine 2004;29:E221–6.
29. Jho HD. Microsurgical anterior cervical foraminotomy for radiculopathy: a new approach to cervical disc herniation. J Neurosurg 1996;84:155–60.
30. Lee JY, Lohr M, Impekoven P, et al. Small keyhole transuncal foraminotomy for unilateral cervical radiculopathy. Acta Neurochir 2006;148:951–8.
31. Saringer W, Nobauer I, Reddy M, et al. Microsurgical anterior cervical foraminot-omy (Uncoforaminotomy) for unilateral radiculopathy: clinical results of a new technique. Acta Neurochir 2002;144:685–94.
32. Snyder GM, Bernhardt AM. Anterior cervical fractional interspace decompression for treatment of cervical radiculopathy. A review of the first 66 cases. Clin Orthop 1989;246:92–9.
33. Henderson CM, Hennessy RG, Shuey HM Jr, et al. Posterior-lateral foraminotomy as an exclusive operative technique for cervical radiculopathy: a review of 846 consecutively operated cases. Neurosurgery 1983;13:504–12.

34. Tomaras CR, Blacklock JB, Parker WD, et al. Outpatient surgical treatment of cervical radiculopathy. J Neurosurg 1997;87:41–3.
35. Tumialan LM, Ponton RP, Gluf WM. Management of unilateral cervical radiculopathy in the military: the cost effectiveness of posterior cervical foraminotomy compared with anterior cervical discectomy and fusion. Neurosurg Focus 2010;28:E17.
36. Clarke MJ, Ecker RD, Krauss WE, et al. Same-segment and adjacent-segment disease following posterior cervical foraminotomy. J Neurosurg Spine 2007;6:5–9.
37. Hilibrand AS, Carlson GD, Bohlman HH, et al. Radiculopathy and myelopathy at segments adjacent to the site of a previous anterior cervical arthrodesis. J Bone Joint Surg Am 1999;81:519–28.
38. Woertgen C, Holzschuh M, Rothoerl RD, et al. Prognostic factors of posterior cervical disc surgery: a prospective, consecutive study of 54 patients. Neurosurgery 1997;40:724–9.
39. Hacker RJ, Miller CG. Failed anterior cervical foraminotomy. J Neurosurg 2003; 98:126–30.
40. Johnson JP, Filler AG, McBride DQ, et al. Anterior cervical foraminotomy for unilateral radicular disease. Spine 2000;25:905–9.
41. Chen BH, Natarajan RN, An HS, et al. Comparison of biomechanical response to surgical procedures used for cervical radiculopathy: posterior keyhole foraminotomy and discectomy versus anterior discectomy with fusion. J Spinal Disord 2001;14:17–20.
42. Chen TY, Crawford NR, Snntag VK, et al. Biomechanical effects of progressive anterior cervical decompression. Spine 2001;26:6–14.
43. Kotani Y, McNulty PS, Abumi K, et al. The role of anteromedial foraminotomy and the uncovertebral joints in the stability of the cervical spine, a biomechanical study. Spine 1998;23:1559–65.
44. White AA III, Southwick WO, Deponte RJ, et al. Relief of pain by anterior cervical-spine fusion for spondylosis. J Bone Joint Surg Am 1973;55:525–34.
45. Bohlman HH, Emery SE, Goodfellow DB, et al. Robinson anterior cervical discectomy and arthrodesis for cervical radiculopathy. J Bone Joint Surg Am 1993;75:1298–307.
46. Winslow CP, Winslow TJ, Wax MK. Dysphonia and dysphagia following the anterior approach to the cervical spine. Arch Otolaryngol Head Neck Surg 2001;127:51–5.
47. Brodke DS, Zdeblick TA. Modified Smith-Robinson procedure for anterior cervical discectomy and fusion. Spine 1992;17:S427–30.
48. Hilibrand AS, Fye MA, Emery SE, et al. Increased rate of arthrodesis with strut grafting after multilevel anterior cervical decompression. Spine 2002;27:146–51.
49. Zdeblick TA, Hughes SS, Riew KD, et al. Failed anterior cervical discectomy and arthrodesis. J Bone Joint Surg Am 1997;79:523–32.
50. Harrop JS, Youssef JA, Maltenfort M, et al. Lumbar adjacent segment degeneration and disease after arthrodesis and total disc arthroplasty. Spine 2008;33:1701–7.
51. DePalma AF, Rothman RH, Lewinneck GE, et al. Anterior interbody fusion for severe disc degeneration. Surg Gynecol Obstet 1972;134:755–8.
52. Ishihara H, Kanamori M, Kawaguchi Y, et al. Adjacent segment disease after anterior cervical interbody fusion. Spine J 2004;4:624–8.
53. Robertson JT, Papadopoulos SM, Traynelis VC. Assessment of adjacent-segment disease in patients treated with cervical fusion or arthroplasty: a prospective 2-year study. J Neurosurg Spine 2005;3:417–23.

54. Yue WM, Brodner W, Highland TR. Long-term results after anterior cervical discectomy and fusion with allograft and plating: a 5- to 11- year radiographic and clinical follow-up study. Spine 2005;30:229–38.
55. Matsunaga S, Kabayama S, Yamamoto T, et al. Strain on intervertebral discs after anterior cervical decompression and fusion. Spine 1999;24:670–5.
56. Pospiech J, Stolke D, Wilke HJ, et al. Intradiscal pressure recordings in the cervical spine. Neurosurgery 1999;44:379–85.
57. Garrido BJ, Taha TA, Sasso RC. Clinical outcomes of Bryan cervical disc arthroplasty a prospective, randomized, controlled, single site trial with 48-month follow-up. J Spinal Disord Tech 2010;23:367–71.
58. Goffin J, van Loon J, Van Calenbergh F, et al. A clinical analysis of 4- and 6-year follow-up results after cervical disc replacement surgery using the Bryan Cervical Disc Prosthesis. J Neurosurg Spine 2010;12:261–9.
59. Anderson PA, Sasso RC, Riew KD. Comparison of adverse events between Bryan artificial cervical disc and anterior cervical arthrodesis. Spine 2008;33:1305–12.
60. Walraevens J, Demaerel P, Suetens P, et al. Longitudinal prospective long-term radiographic follow-up after treatment of single-level cervical disk disease with the Bryan Cervical Disc. Neurosurgery 2010;67:679–87.
61. Barbagallo GM, Assietti R, Corbino L, et al. Early results and review of the literature of a novel hybrid surgical technique combining cervical arthrodesis and disc arthroplasty for treating multilevel degenerative disc disease: opposite or complementary techniques? Eur Spine J 2009;18:S29–39.
62. Herkowitz HN, Kurz LT, Overholt DP. Surgical management of cervical soft disc hernaition. A comparison between the anterior and posterior approach. Spine 1990;15:1026–30.
63. Onimus M, Destrumelle N, Gangloff S. Surgical treatment of cervical disc displacement. Anterior or posterior approach? Rev Chir Orthop Reparatrice Appar Mot 1995;81:296–301.
64. Patil PG, Turner DA, Pietrobon R. National trends in surgical procedures for degenerative cervical spine disease: 1990–2000. Neurosurgery 2005;57:753–8.
65. Wang MC, Kreuter W, Wolfla CE, et al. Trends and variations in cervical spine surgery in the United States: medicare beneficiaries, 1992 to 2005. Spine 2009;34:955–61.
66. Hilton DL Jr. Minimally invasive tubular access for posterior cervical foraminotomy with three-dimensional microscopic visualization and localization with anterior/posterior imaging. Spine J 2007;7:154–8.

Index

Note: Page numbers of article titles are in **boldface** type.

A

Analgesia/analgesics, nonopioid, for radiculopathy, 128
Ankle dorsiflexion test, in lumbar radiculopathy examination, 31–32
Anterior cervical diskectomy and fusion, for cervical radiculopathy, 181
Anterior cervical foraminotomy, for cervical radiculopathy, 182
Anti-inflammatory drugs, nonsteroidal, for radiculopathy, 129–133
Anti–tumor necrosis factor α, for radiculopathy, 132–133
Arm pain, spinal-related, defined, 105

B

Bone scintigraphy, in radiculopathy, 54–55
Bowstring sign, in lumbar radiculopathy examination, 30–31
Braggard sign, in lumbar radiculopathy examination, 31–32

C

Cauda equina syndrome, 172–173
   signs and symptoms of, 172
   surgical treatment of
      options, 172
      outcomes, 173
      timing of, 173
Cervical disk arthroplasty, in cervical radiculopathy management, 182
Cervical radiculopathy
   ESIs for, **149–159.** See also *Epidural steroid injections (ESIs), for cervical radiculopathy.*
   natural history of, 2–3
   surgical treatment of, **179–191**
      anterior cervical diskectomy and fusion in, 181
      anterior cervical foraminotomy in, 182
      cervical disk arthroplasty in, 182
      described, 179
      indications for, 180
      options, 180–182
      outcomes, 183–188
      posterior cervical foraminotomy in, 180–181
Cervical spine, physical examination of, 10–28
   Hoffmann sign in, 28
   Lhermitte sign in, 11
   neck distraction test in, 27

Phys Med Rehabil Clin N Am 22 (2011) 193–199
doi:10.1016/S1047-9651(11)00009-X
1047-9651/11/$ – see front matter © 2011 Elsevier Inc. All rights reserved.

pmr.theclinics.com

Moving?

Make sure your subscription moves with you!

To notify us of your new address, find your **Clinics Account Number** (located on your mailing label above your name), and contact customer service at:

Email: journalscustomerservice-usa@elsevier.com

800-654-2452 (subscribers in the U.S. & Canada)
314-447-8871 (subscribers outside of the U.S. & Canada)

Fax number: 314-447-8029

Elsevier Health Sciences Division
Subscription Customer Service
3251 Riverport Lane
Maryland Heights, MO 63043

*To ensure uninterrupted delivery of your subscription, please notify us at least 4 weeks in advance of move.

Printed and bound by CPI Group (UK) Ltd, Croydon, CR0 4YY

03/10/2024

01040460-0017